GUIDE TO PSYCHIATRIC RESEARCH

Arthur Yuwiler
and
Lennart Wetterberg

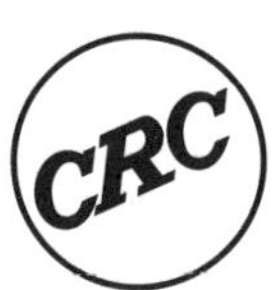

CRC Press

Boca Raton   London   New York   Washington, D.C.

Library of Congress Cataloging-in-Publication Data

Yuwiler, Arthur.
     Guide to psychiatric research / by Arthur Yuwiler and
Lennart Wetterberg.
        p. cm.
     Includes bibliographical references and index.
     ISBN 0-8493-0295-1 (alk. paper)
     1. Psychiatry—Research—Methodology.   I. Wetterberg, Lennart.
II. Title.
     [DNLM: 1. Psychiatry.   2. Research.   WM 20 Y95g 2000]
RC337.Y85 2000
616.89′007′2—dc21

00-039834

Preface

Science is fun — work, but fun. Like art, science forces a recognition of the intricate, detailed, layered, unbelievably beautiful complexity of this miraculous universe that others seldom see. Science and art differ, not in process, despite what some think, but rather in the talent required to make a significant contribution. Whether genius or industrious, everyone in science can help build its soaring mountain of understanding. All that is needed is work, wonder, and thought. And our efforts are cumulative. Every line in every textbook commemorates the lives of dozens of men. The facts endure and become part of human legacy long after the discoverers are forgotten. Indeed, contributing to the body of science is the closest we humans can come to immortality, and there is scarcely any thrill equal to that of being the only person on the entire planet to have discovered something new, of suddenly understanding what was once obscure. Medical science offers yet another thrill. While all of science can eventually contribute to the betterment of mankind, medical science has immediate application. To the general excitement of science is thus added the satisfaction of directly aiding humanity.

This book grew out of seminars on research methodology with medical students, medical residents, and physicians in Sweden, Norway, Boston, and Los Angeles. The intent of the seminars, and this book, has been, frankly, to entice these people into research, or, in lieu of that, to at least make them aware of the salient problems in research and to stimulate their intelligent reading of, and contributions to, the scientific literature.

While this book is intended to introduce psychiatric residents to research, the methodological and moral problems raised are not limited to psychiatry but are relevant to medicine, the medical consumer, and life in general. Science is inductive, and the theories in an inductive system are provisional and subject to change by additional data. Indeed, in the absence of data, all theories are possible; the major function of data is to restrict the number of viable theories. Medical research is no different. Not only is medical research complicated, but medical concepts are also provisional and data dependent. Psychiatry is arguably the most complex specialty in all of medicine, as it involves the mind trying to decipher the mind and attempting to find the mind in the workings of the brain. An appreciation of that complexity may help in understanding why the news can pronounce a cure or warn of a medical danger one day, only to question it the next. Modern science is, after all, scarcely 200 years old … not much time to learn all about a universe that is 5 billion years old. Most of the scientists who have ever lived are living today, and more information accumulates daily than accumulated in a year only a century ago. Moreover, no matter how detailed a medical report, each study samples only a small fraction of the Earth's human population, and that fraction is almost never fully representative of all of mankind. Our knowledge is thus still rudimentary, our concepts provisional. Despite the great similarity between humans, individuals differ so widely in detail that medical practice is still as much an art as a science. It is the intent of this slim book to help push the balance toward science.

The authors

Arthur Yuwiler, Ph.D., is Professor Emeritus, Biobehavioral Sciences, Department of Psychiatry, at the University of California at Los Angeles. He is also the retired chief of neurobiochemistry research, West Los Angles Veterans Administration Hospital, and retired research scientist, U.S. Department of Veterans' Affairs. Dr. Yuwiler earned his Ph.D. in Biochemistry from the University of California at Los Angeles. He was a visiting professor at the Karolinska Institute, Stockholm, Sweden, in 1995, 1996, and 1990, in addition to being a guest collaborator at the National Institute of Health. He was also a visiting senior scientist at the Isotope Department of the Weizmann Institute Rehovot, Israel. Dr. Yuwiler has been a member of the Veterans Administration Basic Science Committee and the Mental Health Research Advisory Committee, State of California, and has served on the editorial boards of the *Journal of Autism and Developmental Disorders* and *Neurochemical Research* and on the scientific advisory board of the Dystonia Medical Research Foundation, as well as serving as chairman of the NIMH Career Development Committee and chairman of the research advisory board of the Dystonia Medical Research Foundation. Dr. Yuwiler is the recipient of the Research Career Scientist Award of the Veterans Administration. He has co-authored another book (*Biochemistry and Behavior*, Van Nostrand, 1964), in addition to writing over 100 scientific articles and contributing nearly 30 chapters to other books. His e-mail address is **ayuwiler@ucla.edu**.

Lennart Wetterberg, M.D., Ph.D., is Professor Emeritus, Psychiatry, the Karolinska Institute, Stockholm, Sweden, and retired Director and Head of the Department of Psychiatry, Karolinska Institute, St. Goran's Hospital. He is also a retired member of the Nobel Prize Assembly of Karolinska Institute in Stockholm. He received his M.D. from the University of Lund, Sweden, and his Ph.D. in Psychiatry and Medical Genetics from the University of Uppsala in Sweden. Dr. Wetterberg has been a Visiting Professor of Psychiatry at the Neuropsychiatric Institute and Hospital of the University of California at Los Angeles, and is an Honorary Member of the American College of Psychiatry. He has organized numerous international symposia, written more than 500 research articles, and edited several books, including *Genetics of Neuropsychiatric Diseases* (Macmillan/Stockton Press, 1989) and *Light and Biological Rhythms in Man* (Pergamon Press, 1993). His e-mail address is **lennart.wetterberg@knv.ki.se**.

Contents

Dedication

We dedicate this to our delightful wives, wonderful children, stimulating colleagues, creative students, the many exciting years of our collaboration, and to the wonders of this unbelievably marvelous universe.

chapter one

Introduction

1.1 Nature of science and medical science

Science is that small branch of general philosophy that takes verifiability as its truth table. That criterion automatically excludes such important aspects of human interest as theology, aesthetics, and ethics which cannot be verified. These are not in conflict with science; they are merely orthogonal to it. By definition, science can say nothing about an omnipotent creator, because, in principle, such a creature cannot be forced to reveal itself. Science can reveal the mechanisms of life but not its purpose, the age of the universe but not why it exists, the process of evolution but not its goal. Similarly, except for requiring absolute truth, science can say nothing about ethics. Whether the strong should rule the weak or the meek should inherit the Earth may be critical to our lives but cannot be verified, although many of the consequences can be predicted. Finally, science can measure physiological and psychological responses to stimuli in the eye of the beholder but not the "intrinsic" beauty of the stimulating object.

Scientists, of course, as humans, have views on these matters, often very strong views. These deserve no more and no less credence than the views of any other intelligent human.

Science has little to contribute to these areas, but all three affect science as a human enterprise. While related, science, medical science, and medicine also differ. The goal of science is to understand. The goal of medicine is to heal. The goal of medical science is to apply the advances of science to the goals of medicine.

While science is devoid of ethics beyond the need for truth, medicine is immersed in ethics and the clinician, like Dr. Arrowsmith in the novel, is often torn between the need to establish the validity of a treatment and the medical needs of a particular patient. In extreme cases, he or she must opt for the latter. Thus, no one will ever make use of untreated controls to evaluate the Pasteur treatment for rabies. However, most outcomes are less dramatic, and comparative procedures are essential to distinguish the useful from the useless.

Despite its limitations, the power of science and scientific medicine is obvious. Both have changed our world. Anesthetics have alleviated pain, antibacterials have eliminated many of the dangers of infection, and new techniques ward off the very deterioration of age. Less obvious than their power is their beauty and excitement. Like artists, scientists are forced to see the grandeur, mystery, and elegance of a universe that most merely take for granted. Few things match the thrill of suddenly understanding a puzzle, of finding unity in seemingly disparate events, of reconciling hidden contradictions, or of being the only creature on the planet to know something. Like Lucretius's river, science is ever changing and never boring. Its practice is exciting, creative, and highly addicting.

1.2   Problem selection and evaluation

1.2.1   Questions

Questions are the blood of science. Devising ways to answer those questions is its heart. Not just any question will do. The requirement for verification means that the questions must be capable of being answered in verifiable form — if not now, at least eventually. This in turn requires that the terms in the question must be operationally defined. Specificity, however, is not always easy. Everyday words for many of our most important experiences are general — love, stress, anger, birds, trees — and until they are operationally defined, their use in studies may confuse rather than clarify. For example, the literature on stress research is a mess because the term is used casually to mean anything from simple discomfort to the appearance of heat-shock proteins. If the definition is specified, the results can be evaluated even though the definition is not necessarily "correct" or universally accepted. As will be discussed later, the use of *Diagnostic and Statistical Manual of Mental Disorders* (DSM; published by the American Psychiatric Association) criteria in defining various "mental diseases" has made possible real comparisons between the results of various studies. Before that, definitions of mental illnesses were often idiosyncratic and comparisons chancy. The fact that DSM criteria have undergone continuous revision, however, indicates that the definitions are neither "true" nor universally accepted. As will be discussed later in Chapter two, the misuse of these criteria beyond the function of communication may not only be misleading but also counterproductive.

A scientist's life, then, consists largely of asking lots and lots of questions and trying to answer the most important. Scientific questions generally fall into two groups: fact finding and hypothesis testing. The first group consists of the newsman's questions of "what" (phenomenon, compounds, symptoms, etc.), "where" (organ, geographic location, cell type, etc.), "when" (after exercise, in winter, after drug), "how much," and "how." Answers to these questions lead to speculations on mechanism and hypothesis. Hypothesis testing generally takes the form of testable "if…then" propositions, the "if" being the hypothesis and the "then" some testable consequence. An example might be the proposition: *If* television violence is a major determinant of social aggression, *then* violence should be less common in rural areas without television relative to adjacent rural areas with television. Note, however, that answering this question rests on answers to a subset of more specific fact-finding questions about the comparability of adjacent rural areas and requires operational definitions of "comparability," "adjacent," "rural," and "violence." A region that does not have television because of social or religious strictures that might themselves influence the frequency of violence, for example, may not be comparable to one without such strictures. Overt physical violence may be different than malicious mischief, etc. Methods development is less directly question oriented and is as much engineering as science.

1.2.2 Sources

If questions are the lifeblood of science, what is their source? Once in science, most questions come directly from ongoing results and the scientific literature. Many questions, however, are prompted by simple curiosity. Følling's curiosity about the funny smell of two children with mental retardation led to the identification of phenylketonuria, and Fleming's curiosity about the clear circles around some molds on a contaminated Petri dish purportedly led to penicillin. New techniques reveal new phenomena and new ways to explore old phenomena at a new level. The term "research" means "re-search, to search again," and this occurs with each new advance in methodology. Magnetic resonance imaging (MRI) now makes it possible to directly ask questions about the anatomy of disease which were very difficult, if not impossible, to answer before. Further refinements may soon allow for examining the *in vivo* status of some metabolites, which, in turn, will allow for better resolution of old questions. New immunological techniques permit quantitation and identification of new peptides whose functions, metabolism, and distributions have yet to be determined, and new techniques in molecular biology reveal both homologies between species and innumerable gene products of unknown function.

Answerable questions also arise from logical extensions of new findings or new approaches. Discovering the coexistence of peptidergic and nonpeptidergic transmitters in the same neuron not only changed the concept of transmitter compartmentation but has also raised a host of still unanswered functional questions about transmitter interactions. The reconceptualization of schizophrenic symptoms provides new ways to examine clinical status and response, while scales fostering consensus on diagnosis enhance comparisons between studies.

Literature conflicts deserve scrutiny as sources for questions. Conflicts arise because of differences in the examined populations, differences in methods, and, more rarely, chance (see Chapter three). Conflicts due to differences in population may provide insight into important subtypes of disease, different etiologies, and unexpected factors influencing disease expression. Conflicts due to differences in methodology may reveal the importance of materials and phenomena other than those thought to be measured. As will be discussed in more detail later, a name is not a thing and many populations defined by symptom expression may not necessarily suffer the same disease.

An even richer vein to be tapped for questions is apparent paradoxes in the literature or incompatible observations. These indicate a need for reconceptualization and are often the source of major advances in science. The digging here can be very hard, however.

Finally, a research problem may be selected for the practical reason that it fits the interests and resources of a preceptor. Under such conditions, selecting a preceptor may be tantamount to selecting a life's work.

1.2.3 *Evaluation*

However selected, a beginning problem, like a beginning love, requires careful attention. It will color all future experiences and may lead to a lifelong association.

A first consideration on looking at a problem is to consider whether it can be subdivided. In science, ignorance is always preferred over confusion. A clear answer to a small question is better than an ambiguous answer to a larger one. Next, can the number of steps in the procedures be minimized? Every step is a potential source of error. Are there ways to maximize the magnitude of the experimental signal and/or decrease background contributions? Can the tools necessary to attack the problem be simplified or improved? Plan how the data will be collected, filed, and statistically treated. Finally, think about the possible ambiguity of results and how to reduce and interpret it.

The overt importance of a problem generally affects funding. Does it weather the test of being a major theory, does it address an important social or health issue, does it extend a technical advance into new fields or resolve a major literature conflict? Measuring the speed of light at right angles to the Earth's rotation was an important experiment by Michaelson and Morley because it tested the ether-drift theory. The use of metallodyes by Ehrlich to treat syphilis was important not only because of its direct medical application but also because it established chemotherapy as a valid medical approach. Loewi's demonstration that material released from a stimulated nerve affected muscle contraction was important because it showed that nerve transmission could be chemical.

Alas, however, the real significance of many projects may not be overtly apparent at the onset. Yalow was awarded the Nobel Prize for her development of radioimmunoassay, work she was initially unable to even get published much less funded. Now the procedure is standard and underlies much of contemporary biology. Pasteur's interest in the souring of wine led to the germ theory of disease. Interest in the sex life of the bacterium, *E. coli*, led to molecular biology. Newton's question of why the moon did not fall when stones and apples did led to the theory of universal gravitation. The moral is, do not let the fads of the moment alone determine the direction of your research. Satisfaction is more important than either reputation or funding. Follow your instincts.

While science is eclectic and can use all talents, an effort should be made to match personal talents with project demands. Some projects are heavily theoretical and others heavily empirical. These attributes change over time, and most projects go through cycles of methods development, fact-finding, hypothesis generation, and hypothesis testing, so the changes may be slow. One individual may find methods development a joy. To another, it is a necessary pain. Data collection may be intrinsically interesting to some and unbearably dull to others. One person may seem to generate a dozen theories a minute while another may not generate one in a lifetime. There are many roads along the path to solving problems, so you may as well find the one most comfortable for you.

Finally, there is also a social aspect to problems. New areas are lonely, often contentious, and always exciting. Older areas are more social, competitive, and generally accepting. With time, the freshly plowed field extends and becomes a highly cultivated farm; what was fresh becomes mundane.

1.2.4 *Literature*

Science is cumulative, and the scientific literature its repository. That repository is now vast and increasing exponentially. The major journals once came out in single yearly volumes. Today a year's publication can fill a full shelf of book space. And the number of printed journals increases daily, as do those on the World Wide Web. Clearly, no one has time to read and digest this growing universe of information, and obviously no one does. The section in Chapter four on how to read a journal is intended to help winnow the wheat from the chaff.

The current literature comes in three forms: papers in journals, reviews, and abstracts. These may be printed but are increasingly becoming available electronically.

The main purpose of a journal article is to present a finding of some importance in sufficient detail to allow for assessment of its meaning and replication of the results. It is the duty of the journal editor and of journal reviewers to assure that it does. How well they do their jobs reflects on the reputation of the journal, and these reputations vary enormously, as will be discussed later. Different parts of the literature take on importance at different stages of a program. In the formative stage, the literature should be read broadly to see if the question of interest has already been answered and to assess the status of the field. During the design phase, the literature is the source for specific experimental procedures and methods, which may appear in articles entirely unrelated to the program of interest. After data collection, the literature is searched again to relate the results with those of others. In between, of course, the literature is read as a source of inspiration and pleasure. Indeed, a chance reading in a seemingly unrelated area has more than once stimulated the development of a research program in a totally different field. Automating weaving led to today's computers, and the sorting of good and bad fruit to CT scans. Serendipity in science and art is not to be eschewed.

Most major journals are now on the Internet and are available by simply searching for the journal name using almost any search engine. Membership in the sponsoring organization or subscription to the on-line version of a magazine is often required to obtain the full text of papers. Abstracts, however, are freely available. General listings of journals can be obtained in hard copy from *Indicus Medicus* or the *Science Citation Index*, or electronically at some of the sites listed below. Most lists are not complete, however, although the *Science Citation Index* site lists some 8500 journals. Some sites, such as Pub Med and the specific journals, provide abstracts or entire articles.

Reviews are useful in acquiring background for a study. Annual reviews are published for many fields such as the *Annual Reviews of Medicine, Annual Reviews of Neuroscience, Annual Reviews of Psychiatry*, etc. Most are comprehensive but are generally six to twelve months out of date at the time of publication. Some review literature reports that are themselves another nine months out of date. Symposium reports, often published in book form, provide more specific information and, while also dated, are usually more current than annual reviews. Still more recent, but also dated, are reviews in current journals. These are usually still more specific and reflect the interpretations of the authors. All of these reviews can be located using various abstracting services, by scanning the table of contents of primary journals, or by computer searches of topic areas. Among the commonly used printed abstracting publications are *Indicus Medicus, Biological Abstracts, Chem Abstracts,* and the *Science Citation Index*. Much of this information is available electronically.

Introductory sections of review articles and their bibliographies can be used as gateways to more specific information. Indeed, judicious reference skipping is often the most efficient route to specific information. The general strategy is to find, perhaps via a key-word search, a very recent article generally related to the specific question of interest and use its reference list to find still more specific references and use those until obtaining the specific information desired. Finding specific information in this manner seldom takes more than six steps, and this application of information theory is the basis for search engines such as the *Science Citation Index* site, which itself is a good starting point.

In contrast to journal articles and reviews, abstracts are intended to summarize findings. They should be used as a guide to the relevant literature, not as a substitute for it. They are the author's interpretation of findings, but authors can be wrong. This is less often the case for journals that are heavily peer-reviewed, but even for these journals a close reading of the actual methods and results sections of a paper is needed to assess the validity of the abstract and, more importantly, the significance of the study. The temptation to substitute the abstract for the paper should be resisted.

The Internet and World Wide Web have enormously increased the ease and convenience of library access. Many on-line abstracting services are now available, and daily more are added. Among the best are the abstracting services of the U.S. National Library of Medicine available in the form of Medline, Grateful Med, and Pub Med which are freely available worldwide. Many journals also publish abstracts of articles electronically, although subscriptions may be required to view the full text. Most of these services permit searches by author, title, journal reference, or key word. Many allow direct linkage to other similar articles. Abstracts and updates on CD-ROM disks may also be obtained commercially.

Convenient as abstracts are, they cannot fully substitute for the journals themselves. As will be discussed later, abstracts are often interpretations not always justified by the methods. Further, few existing electronic abstracting systems extend back earlier than 1963, largely because abstracts and summaries were not routinely required by most journals before then. Abstracting these journal articles anew is time consuming, although some bound compendia of abstracts (*Chemistry Abstracts*, *Psychology Abstracts*, etc.) are issued. Whatever the reasons, much of the earlier literature has been neglected and important discoveries overlooked and/or repeated. A day browsing through the older literature may sometimes save months of work. Library collections of older journals should not be eschewed.

Another great boon to the scientist is electronic communication in the form of e-mail which permits direct communication with and between investigators. Most scientists are willing to share information on procedures, sources, and other technical matters, and e-mail is a good way to seek their help. Because e-mail is viewed and answered at the investigator's convenience, it is much less disruptive than direct phone calls and often more informative.

Medline, Grateful Med, and Pub Med are available from the U.S. National Library of Medicine at:

http://www.nlm.nih.gov/database/freemedl.html

Medical journal links include:

www.sciencekomm.at/journal/medicine/med-bio.html
www.library.ucla.edu/libraries/biomed/cdd/biofbtxtb.htm
www.dlwhe.org/scientific.htm
www.csen.com/scientific-journals/
www.isnet.com/cgi-bin/jrnlst/jlresults.cgi

1.3   Ethics

While science is orthogonal to ethics, ethics impinges on all human activities. Four ethical issues relevant here are the ethics of human research, of animal research, and of scientific interactions and the ethical duties of scientists toward society.

1.3.1   Human studies

Medical science is for the benefit of man, and one of the first strictures of medicine is to do no harm. The clinician-researcher has the difficult task of fulfilling both the role of physician and of scientist, in that order. Accordingly, the first two considerations in studies involving human subjects are "Do the ultimate benefits of the research outweigh the risks for those taking the risks?" and "Is the potential benefit to mankind sufficient to ask someone to take risks for the benefit of others?" Answering either requires some assessment of risks and gains — the risk/benefit ratio. Obviously, the goal is to minimize risk and maximize gain. A potentially dangerous therapy, for example, may be justified to save a life but not to ameliorate a headache.

Subject selection can be even trickier than assessing the risk/benefit ratio. Everyone agrees that subjects in human research should be free, uncoerced volunteers, fully aware of the study and its risks. Sometimes this is much easier to say than to do, however. Informing mentally intact medical subjects is largely a matter of defining unfamiliar terms. The task is much more difficult when dealing with individuals with mental illness, and is especially difficult when dealing with children who are mentally ill or retarded. The moral dilemma is simple. Without study, no treatment can ever be devised. Clearly, that is evil. On the other hand, imposing a treatment on one individual based upon the consent of another, be it legal guardian or parent, may also be evil. Indeed, there really is no general solution to the dilemma. Each case is unique and must be assessed separately. Accordingly, institutional review boards, separate from the investigator, have been developed. It is their difficult task to review assessments of risk/benefit ratios, assure subject anonymity, and assess inclusion and exclusion criteria, recruiting procedures, and adequacy of informed consent. They must also ensure that coercion of any kind, economic or social, is absent, that provisions are made for subjects to withdraw from the study at will and without prejudice, and that subjects receive medical treatment for any untoward effects. The boards should also be acutely aware of the problem. Studies on Alzheimer's disease, for example, must be carried out if Alzheimer's is ever to be treated, but no patient with Alzheimer's disease can ever give truly informed consent. Similarly, unless we are prepared either to let individuals who are mentally retarded or are very mentally ill rot or risk untried treatments, some studies must be carried out. The line is very narrow and great care is needed to tread it.

A standard consent form, then, requires the investigator to:

1. Identify the study as a research study and describe the object and procedure of the study in nontechnical, easily understood language.
2. State that participation is voluntary and can be terminated by the subject at any time without prejudice to subsequent care.

3. Explain how subjects are selected.
4. List the foreseeable benefits and risks of the study to the subject.
5. Ensure confidentiality.
6. List alternative therapies.
7. Explain treatment plans for any untoward effects.

Human protection committees, like all human committees, vary in performance, and it is imperative that investigators do not depend upon them alone to ensure the rights of subjects; instead, investigators should be personally sensitive to moral issues.

Beyond institutionally mandated ethical principles are ethical problems within experimental protocols. A typical example is whether drug tests should compare a new drug against placebo; against another, therapeutically accepted drug; or against nothing. The first alternative controls for the psychological (and thereby physiological) effects of the act of treatment. The second (and most favored by review boards) treats both groups but assumes that the comparison drug, at the dose given, is active against the population tested. The third determines if the drug alters the natural course of the disease.

Each of these approaches poses a moral dilemma. In drug-placebo studies, the advantage of determining if the drug is better than nothing is offset by leaving one group essentially untreated (but also spared side effects). The drug-drug comparison has the advantage that both groups are treated but the disadvantage that neither treatment, for that group, may be better than no treatment. The last has the advantage of assessing the drug against the natural course of the disease but again at the cost of leaving one group untreated.

The ethical problems are further compounded by the dilemma of whether to switch all participants to what appears, at the time, to be the most efficacious treatment. The benefit of not doing so is to obtain further evidence that what seems to be more efficacious really is. The drawback is that some patients, for that study, may not receive the better treatment.

Of course, reality tempers all these considerations. Patients often drop out if treatment does no good or, paradoxically, if it works so well they no longer feel the need for treatment. The statistical problems in evaluating such studies will be discussed in Chapter three. Suffice it to say that the problem of compliance often colors studies.

There are no simple solutions to these problems. What is important, however, is awareness that the problems exist and require consideration. Fortunately, most studies in psychiatric research involve minimal physical risk or discomfort, and most clinician-scientists have sufficient insight into their own motives and feelings to discharge both duties appropriately.

There are many journals on bioethical problems in medicine and innumerable web sites of various quality. One site giving access to many of these others is

aristotle.philosophy.misstate.edu/MedEth/resources.htm

1.3.2 Animal studies

The controversy over experimentation on animals derives from three issues: (1) whether human life is to be valued above other life, (2) whether animal experimentation benefits man, and (3) whether there are alternatives to experimentation on animals.

The first issue is an unanswerable moral question about the equivalence of life. Regardless of theoretical orientation, however, biological machines on this planet need constant input to survive. Except perhaps for green plants and autotrophic bacteria, all creatures on this Earth (including those who raise the question) must kill to eat, be it plant or animal, and most are driven to protect themselves and their offspring. For humans, self-protection and protection of offspring require information, and the animal experimentation needed for either seems justified.

Whether animal experimentation has benefited medicine and humans is an empirical question that can only be answered "yes" based on any fair reading of history and a look at death rates and population growth. Almost all of contemporary medicine derives directly or indirectly from animal studies and their extensions to humans. There cannot really be any question of whether modern medicine has prolonged life and made it more bearable, though there may be a question as to whether we have responded socially to these improvements in such a way as to benefit humans.

The last question is also empirical and must be answered both "yes" and "no." Bacterial, cell, tissue, and organ culture have done much to decrease the need for whole animal studies, although large numbers of animals were required initially to develop these techniques. These cultures have not eliminated the need for such studies, however. The response of the whole cannot yet be fully predicted from the properties of its parts even if those properties are wholly known. Knowing the performance of a carburetor does not alone determine the performance of the car. Even less, do computers eliminate the need for animal experimentation, as many have suggested? Those who know and use computers are aware that the program dictates what a computer does, and if we knew enough about the rules of life to write such a program, there would no longer be the need for it. Computer simulation does not help except to indicate testable possibilities. There are innumerable ways to simulate a phenomenon by processes quite different than those responsible for the phenomenon itself. Robots are not human, and the simulated dinosaurs in movie museums bear no biological resemblance to dinosaurs themselves. A clock, an hourglass, a candle can all be used to measure the rotation of this planet but they are not the rotation of this planet.

While animals must still be used in research, animal subjects deserve the same ethical considerations of necessity, numbers, and maximal humane treatments as do humans. And their use creates the same moral dilemmas as with humans. Nothing is gained if studies are rendered humane to the point of being uninformative, thereby requiring repetition, or of being misleading, thereby leading to damaging therapies. An historical example is the many early neurophysiological studies humanely carried out on anesthetized animals which had to be completely repeated to provide the information on normal neural transactions originally sought, rather than information on anesthesia. Attempts to gain understanding of the processes in trauma such as burns, broken bones, and head injuries in order to provide better therapy pose other uncomfortable dilemmas. Research on such trauma is often as traumatic as the injuries themselves, and the researcher's choice is the terrible dilemma of whether it is better to develop treatments from the results of trial-and-error therapies on afflicted humans or by planned studies on experimentally traumatized animals — truly a dilemma, but one that does not disappear by being ignored. Indeed, ignoring it is itself a choice. As with most ethical issues, good and evil are mixed, and the choice is not clear. What is most needed is an understanding of the complexity of the problem and a tolerance for whatever difficult choice is made.

As one might expect of a moral issue like this, there are many, many views expressed on the Internet. Three sites dealing with the humane treatment of animal subjects are those of the American Physiological Society:

www.faseb.org/aps/animal.html

the American Psychological Association:

www.apa.org/science/anguide/html

and the Canadian Psychological Association:

www.cpa.ca/guide7.html

1.3.3 *Collegial interactions*

Science is an attempt to understand reality. It is also an interdependent collegial activity in which the work of one depends upon the results of others. Clearly the search for reality precludes denying it or substituting fantasy. What is, is, and scientists cannot alter their observations or create others without denying their whole function as scientists, much less as humans. Interpretations of the data can vary but not the data itself. Moreover, the interdependence of science means others will extend or replicate findings. Extensions mean that falsity may cause others to waste a portion of their lives in a meaningless pursuit. Replication means that falsity will inevitably be detected. Any fabrication is thereby not only intrinsically immoral but stupid as well.

Science should be a search for truth and ego independent, but the egos of scientists are no less tender than those of other people. This can pose problems when the ferment of ideas and rapid communication lead several people to have the same idea at about the same time or when the origins of an idea are truly forgotten and treated as original. Both are bound to happen. None of us knows where our ideas come from, and every conversation shapes them differently. It is probably true that some people are more prone to forget than others and, perhaps, should be avoided. On the whole, however, it is probably more productive to assume concurrent conceptions and honest forgetfulness on the part of others and to try to avoid forgetfulness in one's self. Perhaps it helps to recognize that only the data endure and the rest is trivia.

Not only does science beget science, but it also begets collaborations, which grow in size with the need for specialized expertise or equipment. With collaboration comes the problem of appropriate assignment of credit. As mentioned in Chapter four, whenever possible it is better to discuss authorship early rather than late. Authors take responsibility for the accuracy and validity of the results in the paper, and some relationship between the order of authors and the degree of contribution and responsibility should be established. The first name listed on the paper is generally that of the most prestigious author and normally goes to the major contributor. The last name listed is often that of the head of the laboratory who also bears major responsibility for the paper's contents. The placement of other names is usually in the order of their contributions, as well. In some studies where each collaborator contributes equally but differently to the joint study, authorship can be based on lot, can rotate through a series of papers, or can be alphabetical. In such cases, the procedure for assignment should be indicated in a footnote.

Anyone making a major, non-routine contribution to a study should be considered for authorship. This includes the individuals who conceived the study, designed it, devised and/or applied new procedures, interpreted the results, and/or wrote the paper. Assistance of a routine nature — typing, proofreading, carrying out routine assays, etc. — should be acknowledged but generally does not merit co-authorship.

1.3.4 *Science and society*

Scientists owe society an honest, clear recounting of the adventure of science and its results, together with all the "ifs," "ands," and "buts" they would include in recountings to their colleagues. Pronouncement without such qualifications can be misleading. The goal is communication, not sensation. Scientists should help their nonscientific neighbors understand that science is a continuing search for truth and not a repository of *the* truth; that today's conclusions are based on today's data and may change tomorrow; that scientific knowledge is not mystical but is accessible to all. Without such understanding and the information needed to make judgments, many of those outside science are torn between regarding science as the source of the world's ills and seeing science as a repository of information that can solve the world's problems. It is neither and can meet neither expectation.

Similarly, a scientist should resist and protest attempts to hide or distort data for social or political purposes. What is, is, and humans, knowing the truth, have a chance to adapt to it. In any event, reality is impervious to human fiat. As human beings, scientists should make every effort to assure that scientific information is used for the betterment of man and fight against its misapplication.

Scientists are also under obligation to ask reasonably important questions with a presumed significance beyond the fact itself and with some reasonable expectation that the answers will ultimately at least equal the social cost involved. Questions should also be asked in such a way as to avoid or minimize injury or discomfort to any living creature and to be as economical of time and resources as possible.

An excellent discussion of this topic on-line is "On Being a Scientist in Research," put out under the auspices of the U.S. National Academy of Sciences:

www. nap.edu/readingroom/books.obas/

chapter two

Methodology

2.1 Subjects

2.1.1 General considerations and demographics

We humans are very much alike. An estimated 98% of our genome is shared with the chimpanzee, leaving only 2% to account for all that is different between them and us and between ourselves. It is this similarity in biology and behavior that accounts for medicine and society working at all. But individuals are also very different, in both biology and behavior. There are now some six billion people on Earth — six billion individuals. Even a very large study samples only a very small fraction of that total population. While statistics help generalize results from a small sample to a larger one, the mathematical generalization is to populations akin to that studied. But samples are seldom representative of the population of the Earth. Indeed, they are seldom even representative of the population in a particular region.

Obvious factors such as age, sex, and ethnicity can influence basal state, symptoms, and treatment response. They are seldom proportionally represented in most studies. Social isolation has led to many adaptive and maladaptive genetic variants. The Inuit of the north, habituated over centuries to a diet of fish and sea mammals, can tolerate a dietary lipid load that might be deadly for men living in the equatorial belt. The genetic isolation of Askanazi Jews, forced to live for centuries in the ghettos and shtetls of Eastern Europe, has made them vulnerable to many recessive diseases not seen among Sephardic Jews, while neither suffer from the glucose-6-phosphate dehydrogenase deficiency found among Kurdish Jews. Acute intermittent porphyria has a high incidence in Sweden, and sickle cell anemia is almost limited to those of central African ancestry. Genetic isolation has also led to population differences in the activities of many detoxifying enzymes manifest not only in differing responses to alcohol and pharmaceuticals but also to such "natural" common dietary items as peanuts, vegetables, milk, and fat. It is nearly impossible to proportionally represent these populations in any particular study.

More subtle are the effects of cultural and social screening. In countries without a national health plan, such as the U.S. or India, economics plays an important role in who seeks medical attention and when. The poor without health plans usually seek medical care at a later stage of disease than the wealthy. In contrast, those with health care may overuse the system for the medically trivial so the incidence of minor afflictions in the population appears overestimated. A drug study on one population may sometimes not generalize to another because of biological factors and sometimes because of social ones. Social screening or social influences on medical care, however, are not necessarily obviated by universal health care systems. One individual may lose status by becoming a patient in a hospital, while another may gain it. The former will be anxious to get well and leave; the latter reluctant to do so. Culture also affects use. Members of some cultures eschew medical care, some seek it only *in extremis*, and still others use it at the slightest pretext. These cultural factors are not uniform throughout medicine. It may take less discomfort for an individual to consult an internist or cardiologist than an urologist or gynecologist, and while some segments of society would never consider cosmetic surgery, others avidly seek it.

In most of medicine, it is the afflicted themselves who seek help. In psychiatry, to this population must be added those referred by family, neighbors, or by the law. That is, the population entering because of social problems in addition to their physical ones skews the observed psychiatric population. Equally ill but less disruptive subjects or equally ill but protected subjects may simply not be brought to medical attention at all so that the available sample of those who are mentally ill may not be fully representative of the true population. Compounding the problem is the stigma attached to mental illness in some societies, or the reverence given it in others. The effects of these social factors can sometimes be very subtle. As an example, a finding that seemingly confirmed the presence of wider hips and narrower shoulders among male schizophrenics was eventually found to be due to social rather than biological factors. The study was carried out in a state hospital drawing from the lowest socioeconomic status. Femininity was assessed by objective anthropometric bone measures at the hip and shoulder. Initially, the results seemed to indicate a biological or endocrinological abnormality. However, careful analysis showed that patients with a feminine body build, by anthropometric criteria, had higher re-admission rates and longer periods of hospitalization than those with masculine body builds. Admission history showed that this high re-admission rate in turn was a result of police responses to inappropriate or excessive reactions to slights and small acts of aggression. Sociological studies showed a marked hostility by males to feminine traits in the socioeconomic population from which the patients were drawn. Together the data suggested a recycling of that subpopulation of schizophrenics stigmatized with wide hips and narrow shoulders. Such individuals, by their very body build, became unwitting targets for hostility. Their inappropriate responses led to a cycle of hospitalization, treatment, return to the same environments, renewed teasing, inappropriate responses, hospitalization etc. With time, this subpopulation became over-represented in the hospital population at this state hospital which, in turn, led to an accurate, but quite misleading, confirmatory report. The same anthropometric difference was not found, incidentally, in a small private hospital drawing its population from those with a much higher socioeconomic status.

It is this wide individual variance that makes medicine an art rather than a strict science. The mean, developed by science, must be tempered to fit the individual. In addition, because subjects in a study must come from somewhere and are socially screened in the process, demography must be recognized and considered in evaluating the results of each study. Not to do so generates the confusion so evident in the seemingly conflicting medical information reported in the daily press.

2.1.2   Controls

Just as movement is defined by changes in the position of other objects, every study, clinical or not, defines the status of the experimental sample with reference to a comparison sample. Typically, the comparison group is untreated or given an agent other than that being tested. The purpose for doing so is to control for, or equalize, extraneous variables that might influence the results. As a consequence, such groups are generally called controls, and the question then is control for what? In principle, the number of control groups required in a study should be identical to the number of extraneous factors that need be controlled. In some studies, these are very few. In many drug studies, for example, subjects are drawn from a single population and differ only in drug treatment. In such studies, one group is sufficient to serve as control for the other. In longitudinal studies, only a single population is studied, and its status before treatment serves to control for its status after treatment. On the other hand, a search for metabolic concomitants of a disease may require several control populations to account for the effects of such variables as diet, sleep pattern, activity, or emotional condition which may accompany the disease or its treatment. Age- and sex-matched hospital personnel, for example, control, at best, only for age, sex, and humanness. In instances where multiple factors might influence the results, the investigator has only three choices: examine separate populations to control for each of the extraneous variables, normalize environmental variables before the study takes place, or statistically estimate their influence.

Sometimes normalization is too difficult, medically impossible, or unethical. For example, drugs may be required for symptom control, confounding drug effects with those of the disease, or it may be very difficult to equalize population differences in sleeping time. What cannot be normalized in the test population, therefore, needs to be controlled for in the comparison populations. It may be possible, for example, to find other clinical populations treated with the same drug, or who suffer from insomnia, or who have also been chronically hospitalized in the same facility. In some instances, however, despite all effort, extraneous variables can neither be normalized nor controlled. Statistical procedures, co-varying the uncontrolled variables, provide some information on their contributions to the data, but such calculations are heavily dependent on the frequency and variance of those measures in the population studied. If the numbers are small, such estimates can be chancy. In these cases, what cannot be adequately controlled cannot be excluded as contributing to the results, and additional studies may be required. The demographic factors mentioned above apply, of course, to studies where hospital patients comprise both experimental and control populations and when assignment has been random (the importance of random sampling will be discussed later). When hospital populations are compared with external or "normal" controls, however, the methods for recruiting controls may influence their suitability. First, what is their motivation to enter the study? Are controls paid, and if so does such payment select for a particular subpopulation — the poor, the indigent, or college students? If they are not paid, have they volunteered because of altruism, masochism, or external pressures? Are they hospital personnel, differing from patients in education, motivation, and general health? That is, the very fact of volunteering may select for a population which significantly differs from the patient population they are to be compared with. Again, this must be considered in interpreting results.

2.1.3   Patients

2.1.3.1   Sources

As discussed above, the populations available for study vary with the investigator's setting and the patient source. An isolated clinician in private practice may be limited to case studies and longitudinal follow-up of a few unique individuals. Working in a university hospital may allow an investigator a full range of potential studies. Both are valuable. Case studies have often been the first steps in disease identification and therapeutic interventions which were subsequently developed and refined in larger studies. Size alone does not determine quality. On the other hand, population size is important, as we shall see more clearly later, especially when looking for fairly subtle effects.

2.1.3.2 *Selection criteria: diagnosis*

Once a source has been established, subjects and inclusion and exclusion criteria must be defined. The first step in medical management, of course, is diagnosis.

We categorize animals. Often the categories are general. The word "bird" calls to mind a generalized bird, not an ostrich nor a penguin; yet, ostriches and penguins are, of course, birds. Further, the word is not the thing. To call a horse a cow will not provide the family with milk. Both of these kinds of problems exist for diagnosis when etiology is unknown.

Diagnosis seems simple. It is not. It has many functions. In the past, the major role of diagnosis was prognosis — will the king live or die? It directs treatment. It gives access to select social programs. It allows for communication. In many instances, it identifies etiology. Progress in those areas of medicine where etiology is unknown, as is the case for much of psychiatry, has been enormously impacted by failure to recognize these different functions and treat them as though they were interchangeable.

Voltaire said, "Before we argue, let us define our terms." Without agreeing on definition, conversations more often lead to argument than information. A major function of diagnosis is to allow clinicians to communicate. This requires more than a word. "A rose by any other name may smell as sweet," but there is not likely to be consensus on its sweetness if one man calls it a rose and another a cabbage. An agreed-upon definition is also required. Until recently, terms such as "schizophrenia" or "depression" or even "heart disease" were used idiosyncratically, leading to a garbled literature. With time and an understanding of coronary functions, the general term "heart disease" gave way to more specific etiological terms such as "stenosis of the circumflex artery" or "mitral valve prolapse," and progress in cardiology grew apace. Alas, that has not yet occurred in much of psychiatry.

Systems such as the ICD-10 or the *Diagnostic and Statistical Manual of Mental Disorders* (DSM-n) were developed to create some coherence between studies by more or less operationally defining terms. This has allowed clinicians to at least recognize the population being discussed even while disagreeing on the suitability or adequacy of the assigned label. Indeed, the constant revisions of such diagnosis schemes attest to continued disagreements on the validity of the diagnostic words. Whatever their faults and limitations, however, such schemes usefully permit communication and could be termed communication diagnosis.

While a taxonomic reference such as the DSM-n is a great advance over the idiosyncratic use of diagnostic labels, specifying the symptom requirements for a label does not necessarily provide a treatment diagnosis or an etiology diagnosis. The label "299.00 Infantile Autism" may be distinguished from "299.90 Childhood Onset Pervasive Disorder" by DSM criteria, but neither illness has an effective treatment and their etiologies remain unknown. Without an etiology, treatment is generally directed at control of presenting symptoms, regardless of the name given the disorder. A neuroleptic is often given to control acute psychotic outbreaks, whether they are endogenous, due to drugs such as PCP or amphetamine, or in response to an acute infection. Even when the etiology is known, symptomatic treatment diagnosis may take precedence. An antibiotic may be administered without regard to the specific nature of the gram-negative bacteria causing the infection. It is only when the symptomatic treatment fails that the clinician may seek a specific etiological diagnosis while ignoring a general communication diagnosis such as "infection" in the process.

The ultimate identification of a disease requires defining etiology. An etiological diagnosis may or may not define a treatment, as those with Huntington's are acutely aware, but it does provide the possibility of developing a specific treatment. Such a diagnosis is the goal of medical science, just as treatment diagnosis is the goal of medical practice, and it is often the latter's precursor.

The societal diagnosis further complicates an already complex problem by reintroducing idiosyncratic diagnosis back into medical records to facilitate patient access to social programs linked to the communication diagnosis. As a result, the reliability and utility of medical records for retrospective studies, which improved under DSM-IV, are again undermined.

Etiological diagnosis and communication diagnosis often become confused. Generally, etiological diagnosis refers to a subpopulation of those with the communication diagnosis. Thus, the etiological diagnosis of "phenylketonuria" is subsumed under the communicative diagnosis of "mental retardation," and the etiological diagnosis of "stenosis of the circumflex" is subsumed under "heart disease." This confusion becomes devastating in the search for etiology, for it entices the investigator into looking for a correlate of the communication diagnosis. A case in point is the search for the etiology of "schizophrenia." While most agree that schizophrenia is likely the symptomatic endpoint of many different and distinct central nervous system disorders, it is not so treated in fact. Assume for a moment that schizophrenia is the behavioral endpoint of different disorders. Assume that one is the genetic loss of dopamine autoreceptors preventing feedback inhibition; another is a developmental misalignment between hippocampal pyramidal cells making for an improper matching of input to output; a third might be a genetically linked hyper-production of 5HT3 receptors hyperstimulating dopaminergic neurons, thereby increasing dopamine output; a fourth etiology could be an abnormality in membrane structure interfering with second messenger transduction; a fifth could be decreased gabaminergic input to dopaminergic neurons in the nucleus accumbens resulting in their hyperactivity; a sixth might be viral damage to neurons in the reticular formation; etc. Each etiology might disrupt information processing and affective control, and some, by different mechanism, might even act on the same neural substrate. In such an event, however, it must logically follow that those etiologies altering dopamine release differ from those due to viral or developmental interference with neural development. Moreover, the more nearly a measure uncovers one etiology the further it is from the others. Only a small subset of those with the communication diagnosis of schizophrenia, therefore, will express the abnormality associated with a specific etiology. In the current climate, where the communication diagnosis is taken as the etiological diagnosis, even though schizophrenia (or depression or autism or whatever) is assumed to have multiple etiologies, this would lead to abnormalities dismissed as irrelevant.

Indeed, if different etiologies lead to schizophrenia (or autism or depression or personality disorder, for example), congruence between the diagnostic label and some variable is nearly certain to be irrelevant to its etiology and instead due to some properties of the illness or its treatment. It cannot, in principle, lead to the etiology. Indeed, it is arguably the worst possible strategy to use in the search for etiology and the surest road to failure. The communication diagnosis is based on symptom expression, not mechanism. It specifies what is common to the members of that diagnostic population, not what is different, but the difference is critical to etiology. There are numerous examples of biological tests for schizophrenia in the literature. One is the Reigelhaupt test that was developed to detect urinary indoles on the reasonable supposition, one still current, that schizophrenia is due to an abnormality in tryptophan metabolism. The test consisted of overlaying urine onto glyoxylic-sulfuric acid and examining the interface for a purple ring. This was the test used by Hopkins and Cole to first detect tryptophan in proteins. The test proved able, in double-blind studies, to detect schizophrenia in most of the schizophrenic population with almost no false positives. The problem was that it was introduced at the time that Largactal (chlorpromazine) first came into common usage for the treatment of schizophrenia. Unfortunately, Largactal decomposed in strong acid to give a red-purple product. Thus, the test measured the treatment of schizophrenia, not its etiology.

Comparing schizophrenic (or depressive or retarded) populations with controls on some variable, however, is still the near-universal approach to etiology in the psychiatric literature. It is hardly surprising, therefore, that we are still almost as ignorant of etiology as we were at the time of Bleuler and Freud. And, of course, the misuse of the communication diagnosis is not limited to psychiatry but rather occurs in all of medicine when an etiological diagnosis is unavailable.

Alternative strategies will be discussed later. It is important here, however, to note that the name is not necessarily the thing and that while communication diagnosis is necessary for establishing populations, it does not assure etiological uniformity.

The *International Statistical Classification of Diseases and Related Health Problems,* 10th revision (ICD-10), diagnostic criteria can be obtained on-line at:

http://www.who.int/whosis/icd10/index.html

2.1.3.3 *Disease history*

The clinical investigator seldom, if ever, has the opportunity of working with a representative sample of the world's population, nor does the investigator often work with an ideal one. For many studies, an inception cohort collected at, or before, the time of disease expression is such an ideal, as its members are free of the confounding effects of treatment and the ravages of the disease itself. Any other group has, by one means or another, been prescreened in some way and inferences must be tempered accordingly. Individuals who have suffered heart attacks are classic examples of such prescreening. Because only half of those so stricken live to reach a hospital, they represent that segment of the total population spared by some unique factor (anatomy, physiology, disease severity, or simply distance from the hospital) not present in the others. Because they do not represent the full population of those who have suffered heart attacks, results of studies on them must be tempered accordingly.

While heart attacks represent an extreme case, the very nature of most studies selects for populations which limit the generality of results. Consider, for example, the requirements necessary to assess the safety and efficacy of a new drug. First, any study requires informed consent. Subjects should know both the risks and benefits of any procedure. In psychiatry, this automatically excludes all those unable to understand the purpose of and dangers in the procedure or unable to communicate their understanding. Usually these are the very patients most in need of help. Because clinicians will seldom take subjects off an effective medication, many studies inadvertently recruit nonresponders sufficiently motivated to risk a new drug in the hope of getting relief, and studies may also over-represent psychological risk takers.

Because other concomitant medications would complicate interpretation, the examined population should be as free from other drug influences as possible. This leads to a second screening for those acutely ill but previously untreated and/or those chronically ill but taken off ineffective medications. The former are usually young, the latter often older. Medical complications from "recreational" drugs and alcohol are also confounds, and their users are excluded. In the U.S., the use of both is very common among psychiatric patients.

A third factor generally selecting for a younger population is minimizing the risk of testing a new chemotherapeutic agent. Organ dysfunctions generally increase with age, and any organ dysfunction obviously increases the medical risk for any treatment. This is especially true for kidney and liver dysfunctions, as these might interfere with drug clearance.

Finally, pregnant women or women of child-bearing age are also generally excluded for fear of unforeseen tetrogenic effects of the drug. The consequences of this are discussed below.

As a result, even in this relatively simple example, safety and efficacy studies inadvertently select for a relatively young, largely male population primarily suffering either from an acute disease or one unresponsive to current medications. Extrapolating the results to other, more commonly encountered populations requires caution.

2.1.3.4 *Severity*

Wilder's law of initial values points out that it is generally easier to lower an elevated biological variable than to raise it, and, conversely, it is easier to raise a low one than to lower it further. We have all experienced this. It is more difficult for an athlete in a race to increase his speed than to lower it, while someone barely creeping along can more easily go faster than slower. Accordingly, symptom severity influences results by altering the sensitivity of the population to change. A study on antidepressant medications, for example, is more likely to find an effect with severely depressed subjects than with those who are nearly normal if only because rating scales are intrinsically insensitive and have a wider range from high to low than from low to lower. That is, stated differently, sensitivity is inversely related to the magnitude of a measure, especially when measuring instruments are crude. This problem will be more fully discussed later in this chapter. Suffice it to say here that, whether one is doing a study or evaluating a study in the literature, the severity of disease in the population should be considered in evaluating the clinical significance of the results.

2.1.3.5 *Gender*

Most current medical information is on males. This is less a deliberate plot by male doctors than reluctance to put the unborn at risk. Added to this are the experimental complications introduced by the menstrual cycle. As a result, child-bearing women are often deliberately excluded from many studies on new drugs, if only for fear of fetal injury. This leads to the unresolved, and perhaps unresolvable, medical dilemma that avoidance of risk in the experimental stage leads to increased risk in the treatment stage.

The gender composition of studies, therefore, needs to be assessed, and the publication of even small case studies on aberrant clinical responses of women to treatment should be encouraged. Attempts to rectify the informational imbalance by deliberately recruiting women should include long follow-up to assess risk to progeny.

2.1.3.6   Ethnicity

Attention should also be given to the ethnic composition of the population studied and during analysis of the data. Clearly, ethnicity does not label individuals. The variance within ethnic populations on almost any measure is usually greater than the mean differences between them. Thus, while most males are taller than most females, some females are taller than some males. Most Swedes are taller than most Japanese, but a 6'6" Sumi wrestler is 6'6" tall, regardless of the population mean. Nonetheless, as indicated under demography, the activities of liver-detoxifying enzymes, receptor sensitivities, and transduction mechanisms are under genetic influences and evolution has selected for adaptations to local environments. As a result, despite enormous overlap, ethnic differences appear to exist in metabolic responses to disease and treatment, as do social responses. These also need to be recognized and considered in evaluating results.

2.1.3.7   Exclusion criteria

Finally, the applicability of the results of any study is obviously limited to the population studied. Remarkably, this is often overlooked. However necessary, any exclusion criteria limit the universality of the results, but, of course, every study has some explicit or implicit exclusionary criteria. A study on drug response of depressed elderly males obviously requires depressed elderly males, and the results may not be directly applicable to young or old depressed females. Nor should one necessarily expect the results of a study on a population in

Montana to be exactly the same as a similar study carried out on a population in Tokyo.

Most exclusions are explicit in publications. Sometimes, however, they are implicit instead. For example, informed consent for a study on a new drug is unlikely to be sought from, or given by, subjects doing well on an existing medication. Similarly, a study on cognition or motor performance automatically excludes subjects incapable of carrying out the task. In short, look at the methods before you leap to conclusions.

2.2 Procedures

2.2.1 General consideration

Even before beginning a study, a number of considerations will not only clarify the structure of the experiment but also help evaluate the results. First and foremost, what is the real question? The question should be stated as explicitly as possible. Until you know exactly where you are going, it is difficult to pick the easiest route, and it is impossible to tell when you have arrived.

Second, have all the terms in the question been given operational meanings? Many, many important questions are unanswered because they are couched in ambiguous terms leading to ambiguous results. Explicit definition is critical to avoid confusion. For example, if one man stands in the center of circle continually facing a second man who walks the perimeter, has the second man walked around the first man? Without defining what is really meant by the simple term "around," the question is essentially meaningless and ripe for endless arguments. It is like the chicken and egg dilemma. What is an "egg" and what is a "chicken?" Once an egg is defined as embryonic tissue usually surrounded by a shell when laid by a bird or reptile, an answer is obvious, but if an egg is defined as a chick embryo surrounded by a shell laid by a chicken, the question becomes meaningless.

The question "Does stress increase susceptibility to disease?" seems important and simple, but it is not. The words "stress," "susceptibility," and "disease" all must be operationally defined, and their operational definitions temper interpretation of the results. If stress is defined as "anything unpleasant," then the terms "anything" and "unpleasant" must also be operationally defined. If stress is defined by some objective measure such as elevations in glucocorticoid, it should be understood that such a definition would include voluntary "pleasant" experiences, such as riding a roller coaster or sex, as well as involuntary unpleasant experiences, such as breaking a leg or involvement in a family fight. If stress is anything "unpleasant," how is "unpleasant" operationally defined? The magnitude of the change should also be considered, especially if changes are nonlinear. Similarly, "susceptibility" needs to be defined. Is it response to an antigen given to all subjects in the study? Is it the number of reported illnesses in a year? In this case, not only must "illness" be defined, but the experimental groups must also be balanced for their likelihood to report an illness (and of what magnitude?), physical fitness, diet, work site, living conditions, etc. And, finally, is "disease" to be defined as any disturbance, a cold or upset stomach, any illness with a fever, by immunological titer to a standard antigen, or by … what?

Next, consideration should be given to the adequacy of the tools. There is little point in trying to measure either a bacterium or Mount Everest with a ruler. If, as in the illustration above, the level of corticoids or some other biological variable is to be measured, its stability must first be determined. Corticoids, for example, undergo a circadian variation, and levels can sometimes be altered even by the investigator's approach with a needle. On the other hand, blood calcium levels are steady as a rock. As a result, the "when" and "how" of sampling should be included in planning. If rating scales are to be used, what are their sensitivity, validity, and reliability? These will be discussed in greater detail later, but suffice it to say that whatever the tool it must be sufficiently sensitive to pick up the changes expected in the study and in a form that can be used to assess the data. A two-point scale, alive or dead, may be sufficient to assess the lethality of a gun, for example, while more subtle distinctions may be needed to evaluate pain threshold. Similarly, the measure should have some determined relationship to what is being tested, and procedures should be undertaken to assess the reliability and stability of those measures.

Demographics should again be considered. What is the source of subjects, and what factors influence their availability and admission to the study? What are the severity and duration of their illness? The better the populations are defined, the clearer it is for others to assess the relevance and importance of the study.

Who will know the experimental design, and what hand will they have in data collection? The very influence of the physician on a patient, which is so important to therapy, is a hindrance to a scientific study. No matter how well intentioned, investigators cannot help having an emotional investment in a study. As much as they may try to avoid it, the possibility of inadvertently influencing the results cannot be excluded. Those carrying out a study should be blind to the design and the hoped-for results.

Studies are carried out to answer questions, and the broader the answer, the better. Ideally, to maximize generality, studies should be carried out on a random sample of an inception cohort representative of the Earth's population. The design of this ideal study should control for external variables either directly or with adequate control groups. The number of subjects should be commensurate with the expected size of the effect and the variability within the population to provide at least a provisional answer to whatever experimental question is asked. Objective outcome measures of demonstrated validity, reproducibility, and accuracy should be employed, and follow-up should be sufficient to detect long-term consequences of the disease or its treatment.

Clearly, reality is seldom ideal. Instead, an investigator is limited to the available and must temper conclusions accordingly. Inception cohorts seldom walk into the clinic. Rather, most patients come to clinical attention only after developing symptoms and often only after those symptoms are sufficient to impair function. Patient samples are almost never representative of the Earth's population with regard to gender or ethnicity but rather reflect, at best, the local population and local mores. The validity and reliability of measures, especially in psychiatry, are often chancy. Very few studies include long-term follow-up, and sometimes not all pertinent variables can be controlled. Indeed, some are not even recognized except by the results of a study.

The findings of any one study, then, cannot be taken to represent the whole truth but only a portion of the truth, only one piece of the giant puzzle of reality. Literature conflicts should be expected and should be evaluated and understood in terms of the differences in methodologies and populations examined.

Medical studies are roughly divided into those seeking the etiology of disease, those documenting disease incidence and course, and those concerned with perfecting or developing treatment. The following discussion does not attempt to review the vast existing literature in these fields or even to detail all the particulars of different sorts of studies. Rather, it is intended to present an overview of the approach and to point out some of the critical problems to be addressed. Studies on treatment and treatment efficacy have received somewhat greater emphasis, not because they are more important than studies on etiology or disease course, but because the bulk of current psychiatric research is in this area.

2.2.2   Studies on etiology

To know the cause is to be halfway to the cure. Etiological research is perhaps the most rewarding of medical studies and among the most difficult to carry out. The problem of mistaking associations, symptoms, or consequences for disease etiology is persistent. In hindsight, it is clear that impure water does not cause cholera but rather the *Vibro cholera* it often contains, or that the association between damp tropical night air and malaria is not causal but arises because the mosquito bearing Plasmodia breeds in dampness and flies in the evening. Neither was so clear to the astute physicians at the time, however. There is little reason to believe we are any smarter or that today's search for etiology is magically free from the same problems. It is still easy to confound a communication diagnosis with an etiological one, as was discussed in section 2.1.3.2, and it is still difficult to distinguish consequence from cause.

While these problems occur throughout medicine, they are particularly acute in psychiatry. This is largely because behavioral disorders are relegated to other branches of medicine once etiology is clear. Psychiatry, therefore, has become the "neurology of the unknown." Yet, conditions altering behavior — such as neurosyphilis, heavy metal poisoning, physical brain injury, strokes, pellagra, endocrinopathies, psychoactive drugs, fever, and acute intermittent porphyria — provide models for psychiatric research; their very diversity reinforces the likelihood of multiple etiologies underlying the remaining disorders, and they both provide analogies for hypotheses about etiology and examples of successful approaches to their testing.

One lesson to be learned from these conditions is that while it is reasonable to assume that the abnormal functioning of an organ will be manifest in an abnormal output of that organ, the inverse is not necessarily true. That is, abnormal output of an organ may be due to factors outside that organ. The behavioral effects of a high fever can be secondary to an infection in the periphery. *Mycobacterium tuberculosa* attacks the lung but produces melancholia. A deficiency of niacin leads to the "three d's" of pellagra: diarrhea, dermatitis, and dementia. The genetic defect in the structure of the liver enzyme, phenylalanine hydroxylase, which is involved in amino acid metabolism, underlies the mental retardation in phenylketonuria, while defects in another hepatic enzyme, porphobilinogen deaminase, which regulates porphyrin metabolism, leads to the behavioral and biological manifestations of acute intermittent porphyria. That disturbances in peripheral tissues should affect the brain is hardly surprising. Just as the brain mediates events in peripheral tissues, so must the output of those tissues play back on the central nervous system. How else could the organism coordinate its behaviors to meet its biological needs? It may be difficult to do a mathematical problem while distracted by unwanted thoughts, but it is equally difficult to do so with an elephant standing on one's toe. The search for etiology, then, should not eschew abnormalities in peripheral tissues merely because abnormal behavior ultimately represents defective output of the brain.

The great problems in etiological research are in establishing and testing hypotheses. Careful attention to disease onset, time course, symptoms, and familial and environmental associations may contribute to generating hypotheses. To test them, however, requires looking for clinical, biological, pharmacological, or physiological consequences of the hypothesis. Sometimes the clue is simply a biological abnormality of uncertain significance. Each of the diseases mentioned above, now of known etiology, provides a model for the search. In one case, an investigator followed an abnormal color reaction in the urine; in another, dietary eating habits. In all, some abnormality was found to be associated with symptoms, but whether that abnormality was causative or secondary to the syndrome is never clear beforehand. And one can be assured that for every clue leading to a real discovery, there have been dozens of false ones resulting from the disease itself or its treatment. Technological advances increase both the number and kind of variables available for study and sometimes reveal unsuspected relationships and even etiological mechanisms. A germ theory might have evolved even without the microscope, but it is unlikely.

Clinical history and familial incidence underlie hypotheses of genetic contributions to disease. That there are genetic factors in the major mental diseases of schizophrenia and depression has now been firmly established by a variety of familial and twin studies. These same studies, however, also show that, in most instances, other generally unknown factors are also involved. For example, concordance for schizophrenic symptoms among identical twins is on the order of 40 to 60%. The remaining 60 to 40% still needs to be accounted for. It may be due to other genetic influences or to the environmental substate which tempers genetic expression. Even when genetic factors in disease are clear, the site of the lesion and its linkage to symptoms may be obscure. In lieu of direct gene replacement or substitution of the defective gene product, therapy often depends on identifying that gene product and determining how it contributes to symptom expression. Remember, it took nearly 30 years between the time the genetic nature of phenylketonuria was established and its defective gene product identified before finally understanding how that metabolic error led to mental retardation. Indeed, that understanding awaited three critical pieces of information supplied by biochemistry and the neurosciences. The first was the necessary information regarding transport of amino acids into the brain and recognition that excessive blood concentrations of one neutral amino acid (phenylalanine, in this case) blocked the transport of other neutral amino acids into brain. The second piece of information required was that all amino acid must be available before messenger RNA can be translated into protein. The final important piece of information arose from developmental studies demonstrating critical periods in infancy during which protein synthesis is vital for cellular and synaptic development.

Unfortunately, while molecular biology has identified the genetic lesions underlying a number of diseases, for only a few is the linkage between the gene defect and symptoms clear. Acute intermittent porphyria, for example, is a genetically dominant disease, the physical and mental abnormalities of which result somehow from the reduced activity of porphobilinogen deaminase. While this is a terribly important enzyme in porphyrin biosynthesis, its linkage to the symptoms is unclear. Moreover, in Sweden alone there are some 18 known pathological mutations of this enzyme. Another 100 or so have been reported for porphyrias in other populations. Some distinction, then, is needed between the genetic etiology of the disease and the biochemical abnormality leading to symptoms. Moreover, given this, it is not unreasonable to expect unique gene mutations in particular schizophrenic populations. Some may even be errors in gene coding of a single component in a more complex system. For example, the coding may be on something downstream from the neural target. Or, the aberrant coding may not be in the nucleotide sequence coding protein but rather an interfering trinucleotide repeat in the promoter region, as in Fragile X syndrome. The implication of all this is simply that one study may well find a real genetic variant in one population of "schizophrenics" which may not be replicated in another study on another population of "schizophrenics." To establish the etiological significance of a unique gene, then, requires demonstrating its association within a genetically related population, its predictability in identifying those at risk, and, ultimately, identification of the gene product and its relationship to symptom formation. In accordance with Koch's postulate, the gene defect should predict propensity to the disease; while some of the identified population may be asymptomatic, the frequency within the identified population should greatly exceed that of the population free of the gene defect. Conflicts in the literature, therefore, do not constitute *prima facie* evidence of irrelevance.

Acute intermittent porphyria also displays another important phenomenon. The relationship between the severity of symptoms and the gene defect is not invariant. Two individuals with the same genetic defect may vary markedly in symptom expression, even to the extent that one may be asymptomatic while the other dies. This again suggests that other factors besides genetic propensity are necessary for symptom expression. This is a very important and rich area for research.

Many etiological theories of mental disease derive from clinical responses to pharmacological agents and especially to psychotomimetics, neuroleptics, and antidepressants. This derivation is based on the reasonable assumption that anything affecting the clinical course of the symptoms or mimicking the symptoms themselves must be involved in the symptomatic process. However, that linkage can be very indirect. Penicillin, for example, generically blocks cell wall formation by a host of gram-negative bacteria but does not act on the mechanisms of infection. Beta blockers slow heart rate and minimize the effects of vascular stenosis without affecting the mechanisms for plaque formation. And, historically, therapies often preceded understanding of mechanisms. Jenner, noting that cowpox protected milkmaids from smallpox, introduced vaccination well before anyone even dreamed of a virus. As discussed later, many of the most effective pharmacotherapies for psychiatric disorders were discovered by accident during molecular manipulations intended to increase the efficacy of other agents. Nonetheless, their therapeutic efficacy immediately prompted studies on their modes of action in an effort to develop better therapeutic tools and to provide clues to disease etiology. Research demonstrating that neuroleptics derived from chlorpromazine were dopamine receptor blockers while antidepressants, in one way or another, altered synaptic serotonin implicated the monoamines in mental diseases. At nearly the same time, LSD and many hallucinogenic agents were discovered. Some indoles, such as bufotenin, psilocybin, and even LSD itself, resembled serotonin, while mescaline and amphetamine were catecholamines, such as norepinephrine and dopamine. The dopaminergic theory of schizophrenia and the serotonin theories of depression, schizophrenia, and mood disorders were derived from these and subsequent studies. In a parallel fashion, more recent glutaminergic theories of schizophrenia derive from evidence that hallucinogens such as phencyclidine act on glutaminergic NMDA-receptors.

The various transmitter hypotheses are still relatively vague and general. They will become stronger as the anatomical basis is clarified and the aberrant receptor subtypes or their downstream components are specified. Clearly, if lesions in specific transmitter systems are the underlying etiology of some of these illnesses, those afflicted should show greater therapeutic response to agents specific for some aspect of that transmitter system, be it a particular receptor subtype, some transmitter interaction, or some cotransmitter. Increasingly, however, it seems unlikely that any single transmitter lesion is entirely adequate to explain all symptom expression in major psychiatric diseases. The anatomical linkage between transmitters, the interactions between transmitter systems, the complexity of each transmitter's receptor subtypes, the coexistence of peptidergic and "classical" transmitters, and the intricate cascade of events initiated by receptor activation suggest that none of the current hypotheses need to be mutually exclusive and that, indeed, there are likely lots of ways to produce changes in mentation and behavior. Newer drugs, acting on new sets of transmitter subtypes, have suggested that at least some forms of mental disease require a treatment other than simple blockade of D2 receptors. There are likely multiple roads to Rome.

Anatomical support for developmental disruptions in the etiology of mental illness derives from studies at both the microscopic level and at the functional levels of positron emission tomography, computerized tomography, magnetic resonance imaging, and multiencephalography. From immunological data on animals and humans have come proposals that some of these developmental disruptions are secondary to prenatal bacterial or viral infections. Presumably, those so afflicted would show exacerbated symptom expression at the time the afflicted region becomes functionally important. In addition, such individuals might be expected to be relatively unresponsive to transmitter-directed therapeutic agents.

Sociological hypotheses of the genesis of psychiatric illnesses derive from familial incidence, but the search for a hypothetical schizophrenogenic parent or environment cannot be seriously undertaken until the "schizophrenogenic" component is operationally identified. This is not yet the case, and the vague reference to an undefined "stress" is inadequate to examine the proposition.

While the etiology of a metabolic disease is most often discovered by the simple detailed case studies of a few select individuals, verification usually requires demonstrating a linkage between symptom expression and the hypothesized etiological agent in a random population or one selected to resemble the afflicted population in all particulars except the provocative agent in question.

2.2.3   *Studies on disease course*

Documenting the natural course of disease was once a major area of medicine and the key to prognosis. In those areas for which there are effective medical treatments, emphasis has shifted from disease course to the two extremes of identifying possible precipitating influences and predromal symptoms to assessing the long-term consequences of the disease and its treatments. Nations vary widely in the ease with which such studies can be carried out, partly as a function of the ease of access to medical care. Defining prodromal symptoms and assessing prognosis depend upon an inception cohort. Any other population is suspect of not truly representing the diseased population but rather that subset in need of, and able to obtain, medical attention. A similar problem exists with retrospective studies using medical records which may be additionally complicated by changes in disease criteria and identification over time. This is a particular problem in psychiatry, in which, until fairly recently, diagnosis was almost idiosyncratic.

The long-term consequences of disease or of its treatment are of obvious medical importance and are easily overlooked when attempting to maximize medical economics. Immediate side effects are relatively easy to detect and guard against. Long-term consequences of treatment or long-term changes in clinical state are more difficult to define, and the difficulty grows with time and the consequent accumulation of other possible contributing influences. This is evident today in regard to the decades-old fight to evaluate the dangers of "recreational" tobacco, alcohol, and drugs. The comparatively long life span of humans also complicates the assessment of long-term effects of any agent. It is difficult to know what effects a treatment introduced today will have 30 years down the line, and most are understandably impatient to wait 30 years to find out. Studies on shorter-lived animals such as mice and rats are used instead to provide some clues, but rodents are not humans, clues are not certainty, and

30 years are still required to reveal what the effects will be at that time.

2.2.4 Studies on treatments

2.2.4.1 Drugs

2.2.4.1.1 Herbal medicines. Herbal medicines were probably used to treat disease even before recorded history. Animals have to eat, but plants do not like to be eaten. To avoid such a fate, plants have become marvelous chemical factories evolving a few external defenses, such as spines, but lots of internal ones, also, such as toxins, fungicides, pesticides, bitter-tasting compounds, and, of course, the anthocyanines, carotinoids, auxins, and other compounds that give them color and drive their life cycles. An omnivore such as humans can eat virtually anything that crawls on the Earth, from ants to rattlesnakes, but relatively few plants. Toxicity itself indicates pharmacological activity. Often, with proper dilution and usage, and in lieu of alternatives, that pharmacological activity can be of medical use. Indeed, plants have given, and are giving, much to our pharmacological armament, ranging from aspirin to digitalis.

A major problem with herbal medicines, however, is evident to every wine connoisseur. Grapes from the same plants, in the same soil, produce great wine one year and virtual vinegar the next. That is, the chemical composition of the product of even the same plant is subject to the vagaries of temperature, moisture, soil bacteria, and countless other uncontrolled and unrecognized variables. Without identifying and quantifying the active ingredients in an herb, rational dosage is impossible. Indeed, the effort involved in natural product isolation and production of active components is largely driven by the need to control dosage. A gram of vitamin C is a gram of vitamin C, whether a man or a plant synthesizes it. And dose can be critical. Botulinum toxin, appropriately applied in low doses, may control the blepharospasm of dystonia. At a higher dose or administered differently, it will kill. Only a moment's thought is needed to conjure up other examples.

The coupling of human variability with the myth that "natural is not dangerous" poses another problem in herbal treatments. Of course, the problem of human verifiability exists with any product, natural or synthetic, but while most acknowledge that prescription drugs may have side effects, many forget that "natural" products do, too. One child may be allergic to peanuts, a natural product, while another may dote on them. Aspirin, derived from a natural product, causes ulceration in one person while another takes it daily for platelet control. It takes little thought to dismiss the notion that "natural is not dangerous." The alkaloids in "natural" toadstools kill. Botulism is "natural" but deadly. No one in his right mind chews oleander leaves, etc. To the extent that herbal medicines are physiologically active, at least as much caution should be exercised in their use as is exercised with pharmaceuticals. Fortunately, most herbal medicines are used at concentrations well below their physiological potential. That may not make for the most effective pharmacology, but it is good business.

2.2.4.1.2 Chemotherapy. It was Ehrlich's brilliant conceptual wedding of the toxicity of arsenic, nitrogen's cousin on the periodic table, to the specificity of the N=N linkage in azo dyes that gave us salvarsan and began chemotherapy — the attempt to rationally design therapeutic drugs. That his driving hypothesis was wrong is irrelevant. Indeed, until very recently, the history of medical pharmacology is as much a litany of accidental drug discovery as rational drug development. The specificity of azo dyes led Domgask to try the dye protonsil, soluble as a bacteriostatic agent. Its efficacy changed medical history, especially when it was found that its potency lay in its sulfanilamide moiety. The resultant sulfa drugs turned the tide against infectious disease. Subsequently, penicillin, streptomycin, and related compounds again reinforced the medical value of plant products. Today, growing information on enzyme and receptor structure and function is providing a whole new rationale for drug development and medical pharmacology.

In contrast to the semi-rational development of pharmacological interventions in most of medicine, advances in psychiatric pharmacology have until recently been even more haphazard and fortuitous. In large part this reflects our ignorance of the workings of the human brain and how the operation of this organ is transmuted into the ephemeral products of thought and emotion. Chlorpromazine, the first neuroleptic, revolutionized the medical treatment of psychiatric disease but was the fortuitous result of trying to make a better antihistamine than promazine. Indeed, until recently, chemical pharmacology at all levels consisted largely of manipulating the structure of therapeutically active molecules. This effort was driven in part by a scramble for patents and, in part, by the wish to enhance drug efficacy and specificity. Thus, iproniazide, the first antidepressant, was developed as an analogue of the antitubercular agent, isoniazide. Its antidepressant properties were noted when the mood of tubercular patients improved even more quickly than their health. Substituting a C=C in place of S in chlorpromazine resulted in the first tricyclic antidepressant rather than simply a better chlorpromazine.

This general approach of molecular iterations has begun to change in more recent years. While molecular manipulations still go on, the targets now are receptors and animal models thought to mimic the end behaviors rather than simply two-dimensional alterations of active molecules. The adequacy of the animal models and the linkage between receptors and behaviors are continuing matters of cumulative investigation in which the properties of new compounds, therapeutic or not, and new models help clarify the biology of the mind.

Clinical trials. Establishing the clinical utility of a new drug is a long and costly process. Each country has its own procedures and criteria. Currently, in the U.S., a drug must go through three phases before receiving official approval for clinical use. Phase I consists of a human study to establish human safety and appropriate dose schedules. Phase II has the purpose of establishing whether the drug has clinical efficacy. Phase III has the goal of assessing the efficacy of the drug relative to other available drugs. All three of these phases depend on tests that are adequate to their tasks. These will be discussed later, but it is important to note that the tests used must be sensitive, appropriate to the specific goals of the study, and verifiable.

Phase I. All beginnings are difficult, and Phase I studies in addition contain some elements of danger. Although animal studies on safety and dosage help guide human studies, rats are not human, either behaviorally or biologically. Establishing safety and dosage in humans is therefore necessary as a preliminary to clinical usage. The two major goals of Phase I studies are to establish safety and appropriate dosage; questions of efficacy are secondary.

The safety issue requires excluding from the population to be tested those who might be at risk in the study. Usually this means excluding anyone with liver or kidney disease, women of child-bearing age, and, depending on the drug, those with other organ diseases as well, a restriction that often excludes subjects over 65. In addition, Phase I studies, like all human studies, require informed consent, thus anyone under 18 years of age is excluded. Also, because safety has not been established, patients are likely to volunteer only when their symptoms are particularly disturbing, when alternative therapies are unavailable or ineffective, or when they are paid in one form or another. As a consequence, experimental populations in Phase I studies often are heavily weighted with healthy, normal controls, even though the drugs will later be used on patients and the two populations may differ somewhat in drug detoxification and utilization. (The possible problems with normal volunteers in studies like these have already been discussed in section 2.1.2.) Phase I results, therefore, should be viewed as critical guides but not necessarily established dictum.

The second goal of Phase I studies is to establish appropriate dosage. In theory, appropriate dosage usually means the minimum dose producing the desired clinical response with minimal risk of side effects. Because of the wide variance in human biology, the effective dosage is the median or average dose needed, and the variance in dosage can be quite large. The lower limit of the range is often about half the dose needed to gain the maximal clinical effect, and the upper limit is the level at which 5 to 10% of subjects suffer side effects. Tolerance for side effects, of course, varies somewhat with the disease, its severity, and the general health of the test subject. The dosage and side effects tolerable to prevent death may be clearly excessive for the treatment of a mild headache. The dosages affecting normal controls, further, may widely differ from those effective against a diseased population. A classic example is chlorpromazine, which, at doses putting a normal control to sleep, may have no effect on the psychotic episode of an acutely ill schizophrenic.

To establish safety, laboratory tests assessing the status of vital organs and reliable measures of pathology such as clinical screens are needed. To establish efficacy, the tests of pathology must be sufficiently sensitive to detect subtle change. These may be both biological (EEG, EKG, etc.) and behavioral (test of mental or physical performance and mood.) As will be discussed below, the problems of validity, reliability, and sensitivity of testing in psychiatry are not trivial.

Phase II. Once issues of dosage and safety have been addressed, the next task is to evaluate efficacy. The population for such studies should be randomly assigned, free of previous drug treatments, representative of the general patient population, and homogeneous with regard to symptoms. Because efficacy is the issue, the population must consist of patients and the duration must be sufficient to provide a fair estimate of clinical response. Ideally, long-term follow-up should also be carried out to assess the long-term effects of treatment. Finally, efficacy should be evaluated against placebo.

This, again, is the ideal. Seldom, if ever, are these requirements met. First, no site is representative of the Earth's ethnic and gender populations. Multicenter studies, sampling a much larger and diverse population than is available at any single site, can better approximate at least the national population mix and are preferred to a single-site study. The resultant problems of consistency and reproducibility in multicenter studies will be discussed later.

Population. Even multicenter studies do not often adequately represent the Earth's populations. Representation is narrowed further by the necessary exclusion criteria eliminating those with organ disease which might compromise the study and, of course, often women of child-bearing age. Also, because it is medically unethical to switch a patient who is responding to one drug to another of unknown efficacy, nonresponders are generally over-represented in some studies in Phase II testing. On the other hand, there may be pressure for pharmaceutical companies and investigators to recruit good responders. The selection criteria are thus of considerable importance in evaluating the results. A slight positive effect of the drug on nonresponders may, in fact, be more impressive than a standard response by responders.

Placebo. Clearly, one cannot tell if something is better than nothing, especially if the effect is marginal, without comparing it to nothing. Placebos are often assumed to be that nothing, but there are both ethical and practical problems in their use. First, placebos are really not inert, and both positive and negative responses have been reported. Because the mind runs the body, this finding should not be surprising. People have died from merely hearing bad news, although nothing has physically happened to them. A sound in the dark can set the heart racing, although nothing threatening has occurred. Movies and novels arouse fear, love, and hate, even though the events depicted are not real and do not in any way alter the viewer's circumstances. Indeed, in some instances, as much as 40% of the therapeutic response to some agents in some people may be a placebo effect. Indeed, in some instances, a placebo has been shown to have a therapeutic value with lesser side effects than therapeutically active compounds. While it is generally assumed that placebo effects occur early and are of short duration, this may be more of an assumption in some instances than a reality. In any event, placebo responses need to be reckoned with. Beyond their influence on response, placebos raise a moral problem. They are not intentionally therapeutic; therefore, it seems medically impermissible to foist them on patients seeking therapy. Yet, without a placebo comparison it is difficult to assess efficacy.

A third problem with the use of placebos is in recruitment. There is a moral and practical need for informed consent in any human study. Patients may understandably be reluctant to risk inclusion in a placebo group rather than in a presumably therapeutic one when they are in need of help. To avoid this moral dilemma, some investigators have tested for, and removed, placebo responders from the experimental population. This leads to two problems. First, it may exaggerate efficacy. A 2% increase over a 30% placebo effect is less impressive than a 2% increase over baseline. Second, placebo responses within an individual may not always be consistent. Alternatives are to carry out a within-subject "before/after" analysis or to carry out a semi-Phase III study comparing the agent in question against another of "proven" therapeutic value. Of course, if the tested compound is better or equal to the presumed standard, the question of whether either is truly effective against the tested population is open. This might be the case, for example, if the tested population consisted of drug nonresponders.

Subject selection: randomization. Phase II results should give clinicians some idea of the efficacy of a new treatment for their patients as compared to existing treatments. This will be the case when the results are representative of the general population and the treatment groups are selected without bias, which is more likely to occur if the patients are randomly selected from a very large population. In addition, most statistical procedures for analyzing group differences and treatment effects assume random bell-shaped Gaussian distributions of measures. For both reasons, then, group assignments should be randomized. If they are not, either other statistical procedures must be used or the generality and validity of the comparisons are compromised.

Randomization is more than a sequential assignment of subjects to groups as they come out of admission. Rather, it is really random assignment. It requires something like numbering sequential subjects from 1 to N and assigning them to groups in accordance with some random number system, usually a random number table as found in most statistical texts, or a computer-generated random number sequence. In such processes, numbers larger than the total sample size are ignored as are numbers already taken.

The matter becomes further complicated if different groups are considered. For example, if two groups of 20-year-old male depressives are to be compared for response, then only two random groups need be involved. However, if the males and females within the group are also to be compared, then the number of randomized groups increases to four. If those with or without hospitalization are to be compared as well, then the number of randomized groups jumps to eight. That is, if the population is stratified into other groups, then the number of randomized groups that need to be selected is two raised to the power of the number of groups. Obviously, the more stratifications, the larger the required populations and the greater the logistic problems in acquiring the requisite population.

Subject selection: matching. As any gambler knows, random flips of a fair coin will eventually produce an equal distribution of heads and tails. What many gamblers do not believe is that coins have no memory and that each flip is independent. In the short term, runs of heads and tails are likely to occur but, using an honest coin, the flip after 1000 tails still has an equal chance of being heads or tails. The runs pose a problem, however. When the number of subjects is very small, true random selections may lead to uneven population distributions. This problem diminishes with N. As an extreme example, suppose one wanted an equal distribution of males and females in two groups and the population consists of just two males and two females to be randomly assigned into the two populations. There are eight possible pairings of mixed groups, and four pairings of single-sex groups, or a ratio of 2:1. If the population consists of three of each sex, the final distribution is 18 mixed couples and 12 same-sex couples, or 3:2. The ratio is 4:3 if there are four of each sex and diminishes further with an increased N.

The same pattern is also true if, as more likely, the numbers are uneven. Thus, when populations are small, random assignment may not represent gender (or any other dichotomous variable which may be critical to the outcome measure) equally between populations, and the results from such a study must take this into account. Although such a skewed population distribution may preclude a clear conclusion in a small study, the randomization does permit pooling. That is, if the population is really randomly selected, the clinical trial well conducted, and the methods and results clearly presented, the study can be pooled with others to provide results on a larger population. Such meta-analysis is more difficult if the populations in each study are more idiosyncratically chosen.

An alternative to randomization is matching, which is used, of course, when populations are so small as to produce uneven distributions of critical variables. It should be noted, however, that each variable that is matched acts to successively screen the population from which the sample is drawn. Not only does this skew the sample away from the true population but, again, the more matching variables that are required, the larger the population must be. Because limited population size is often the reason for matching, the use of many matching variables is self-defeating and only the most critical should be considered.

Phase III. The goal of Phase III studies is to establish the efficacy of a proposed treatment relative to other established therapies. In many ways, Phase III studies are easier to carry out than Phase I or II studies because issues of both safety and efficacy have already been established. There are fewer moral conflicts. Also, because the proposed drug is efficacious, recruitment is much easier, especially from subjects either refractory to existing medications or suffering from their side effects. Indeed, Phase III studies, in one form or another, fill the literature; however, because of vested interests in the results, the methodology of these studies requires close attention and caution is often necessary when evaluating them.

Many subjects for Phase III studies have been exposed to alternative drug therapies in the near past; for them, a drug washout period is required before beginning another treatment. The primary purpose of this period is to prevent drug interactions and mistaking the therapeutic actions of the old drug from the properties of the new one. In practice, the duration of this drug-free period is often an uneasy compromise between the need to avoid mixed drug effects and the needs of the subjects. Sometimes the washout period is converted into a placebo period to both identify placebo responders and provide an independent baseline. Sometimes it is simply a drug-free period. In both cases, close clinical attention is required to detect any recrudescence of symptoms requiring immediate reinstitution of treatment.

The pharmacokinetic properties of the treatments may also affect the duration of the drug-free period. Many psychoactive drugs are organic bases which deposit in lipids, and their complete clearance from the body is slow. In addition, many are detoxified by similar enzymes, the activity of which may be inducible. As a result, one drug may alter the normal rate of catabolism and elimination of a second drug. Again, the time for these effects is variable, and some persist long after blood levels of the agent are no longer detectable.

All this dictates that, ideally, the washout period should be a prolonged one. On the other hand, the longer the drug-free period, the more likely it is that subjects will be lost to the study due to either increased symptomatology or withdrawal of consent. The subject, after all, no matter how altruistic, is seeking relief from symptoms, and the physician's primary goal is to help produce that relief. There is no satisfactory solution to this dilemma beyond suggesting that the drug-free period should be as long as feasible, up to about a month, but the rule of thumb is often two weeks or less.

Phase III studies come in three flavors: open label, single blind, and double blind. The degree of trust in the meaning of the results should be in the reverse order: double blind over single blind over open label. An open-label study is one in which everyone is aware of the treatments and is susceptible to the enthusiasms of the staff. Indeed, in general, the results of open trials tend to cluster on the high end of efficacy. They are carried out because of existing uncertainties over dosage, the nature and magnitude of the therapeutic response, the nature of the responsive populations, and the uncertainty of idiosyncratic side effects. Open-label studies are a common and, indeed, necessary, preliminary step to subsequent better controlled studies.

Single-blind studies are ones in which the investigator alone knows the nature of the treatments. While still subject to experimental bias, this type of study allows for clinical responses to adverse drug effects and for individual adjustment of dose.

Of the three procedures, the results of double-blind studies are least likely to be influenced by experimenter bias. In these studies, a third party not involved in treatment, data gathering, or analysis controls the assignment of medication. The investigator, of course, still controls the inclusion and exclusion criteria which define the population studied and selects the measures to be used to identify the specific criteria to be investigated. While these actions circumscribe the results, they do not affect replication.

The first trial of a drug is often more promising than later trials due to the so-called miracle drug effect. In the general mind, this often-seen phenomenon is assumed to demonstrate investigator bias. Most often it does not. Most often it is the coupling of our continual search for signals large enough to be seen over the general noise of the universe with a population particularly sensitive to a therapeutic agent. Given a random distribution of drug sensitivity, someone somewhere will, by chance, have access to a population particularly responsive to some agent. That investigator will see a clear therapeutic change well above the therapeutic noise level and report it. Those who try the agent with less favorable populations will see only a more modest change and may scarcely bother to publish. One great advantage of electronic publishing, as was discussed previously, is to facilitate publication of negative and mildly positive data and thereby provide a clearer picture of medical interventions than is now available. What is often neglected when considering this phenomenon, however, is that recognizing that the hypersensitive population is hypersensitive for some reason — pharmacokinetics, receptor numbers, or distributions, or perhaps even etiology — is a clue worth following rather than ignoring.

Study design. Clinical trials are usually carried out in one of three major designs: longitudinal, parallel, and crossover. Each has its advantages and problems.

Longitudinal. The basic design of a longitudinal study is to use each individual as his or her own control and to compare clinical states before and after treatment. This is probably the most common design for Phase I and Phase II studies; it is less common for between-drug comparisons in Phase III. The basic hypothesis underlying this design is that, over the time of the trials, clinical response without intervention will either fluctuate or deteriorate but not significantly improve. Further, it assumes that there will be no learning effect of the instruments used to assess clinical change and that the tests themselves are stable over time. The question of establishing and maintaining the reproducibility of test results is discussed below. In general, these assumptions usually hold, although adaptation to measures, especially some psychological measures, should be considered.

The repetitive data obtained in longitudinal studies are best handled by statistical programs designed for repeated measures rather than those such as the Student T-test or a simple analysis of variance designed for group comparisons. Trends in the data derived from longitudinal studies, even when not themselves statistically significant, can form the basis for larger scale studies.

Parallel. Parallel group designs are the most popular in psychiatry, partly because they are so adaptable. As the name implies, the parallel group design maintains two or more groups in parallel throughout the study. There are many variations of this simple theme. In one, the treatment is varied between groups. In another, the groups are varied but the treatment is not. For example, in Phase I, the efficacy of a new drug or treatment might be examined by treating one population with the drug and treating another concurrently in parallel with a presumed ineffective treatment or with placebo. In Phase III, one treatment would be compared with another established treatment. Still another design might be to compare the efficacy of the drug on young vs. older patients or males vs. females. The number of comparison groups, it should be noted, is not limited to two.

In general, this design does much to control for factors such as adaptation, seasonal effects, and environmental perturbations. It is also easier to keep testers blind to treatments; however, it does not ensure tester blindness. Indeed, the more effective the treatment and the greater the difference between the treatment and placebo groups, the more difficult it is to keep the clinical staff from correctly guessing the treatment paradigm. One way of ameliorating this is to compare one drug or treatment with another active drug or treatment rather than with a placebo or ineffective treatment. Even then, maintaining the blind is most effective and most needed when treatments are marginally different. It is impossible to maintain the blind when a truly effective treatment is used. That is, if drug X seemed to "cure" schizophrenia, there would be little question that staff would identify the treated.

The great utility of the parallel design is paid for by its high demand for subjects; the more groups examined and the more variables in each to be matched, the larger the source population must be.

Crossover. The crossover design squeezes a parallel design into a longitudinal one. Like the longitudinal design, crossover design is more conservative of subjects than the parallel. Rather than comparing changes between populations, where the number of subjects required is the product of the number of treatments and the number of groups required to control for critical variables, the crossover design assesses changes within individuals so that populations are their own controls and the number of groups is determined by the number of treatments. In most cases, the design is such that half the population receives treatment A, while the other half receives placebo B. After some time, the treatments reverse to yield AB, BA. In some cases, comparison is made between two active compounds, A and C, and a no-treatment group, D, is also included. In this instance, the groups would be AB, BA, AC, CA, and DD. What is measured in this case is the difference in magnitude of the effects of treatments A and C compared to the untreated group, D. Obviously, the sign of the difference changes in accordance with treatment order. An alternative design is ABCD for one group and BCAD for another, permitting some direct comparisons of the drugs' relative effectiveness relative to baseline.

In most instances, a no-treatment or drug-free period is also introduced at the beginning of the sequence to minimize the influence of any preceding treatments on the results. Treatment periods for A and B (and C) need not be the same, but they should be constant. Because of overlap and the concurrence of treatments, it is usually easier to keep staff blind to treatment than is the case for parallel group designs. Included also in this paradigm are replicate ABAB (and their counterpart BABA) designs, which are used to efficiently and convincingly replicate findings on the same population.

The virtues of the crossover design are rather obvious. Individuals serve as their own controls, the data are automatically replicated (thus, any effects of treatment are convincing), the number of treatments does not multiply the number of subjects, and concerns about contributions from extraneous variables are minimized. What is gained in numbers, however, is paid for in time and logistical complications. Crossover studies generally take longer than parallel studies and are much more sensitive to missing data and dropouts. Because the longer the duration of a study the larger the dropout rate to be expected, the increased duration of crossover studies carries a double penalty. Further, dropout rates increase if treatment is effective and placebo is not. Not only are patients unlikely to acquiesce to change from a treatment that elicits improvement to one that might not, but ethical issues are also involved. Such issues are somewhat ameliorated in designs alternating presumed effective treatments.

Besides these factors, the design requires that the effects of treatment be reversible and that termination of treatment leads to an immediate or rapid return to pretreatment levels. The design is not applicable to conditions where treatment produces enduring changes, as this precludes a post-treatment return to baseline within any reasonable time period. This is the case, for example, with antibiotics, which cure an infection so there can be no return to baseline, or for antipsychotics, where several weeks of treatment are required to produce a clinical change and behavioral and some biological changes often persist for long periods after drug withdrawal.

2.2.4.2 *Psychotherapy*

The clinical use of psychopharmacology is intended to restore normal function to an abnormally functioning brain leading to the normal operation of mind. Its intended purpose is no different than the medical use of organic nitrates in cardiology to relax coronary vessels and increase blood flow to the otherwise abnormally functioning heart. Neither therapy is entirely successful and neither cures, but both represent great advances in the medical treatment of disease.

In contrast to other organs, however, brain function is also susceptible to modification by the non-chemical interventions of sensory input. Such changes are considerably more regionally specific and functionally selective than today's relatively crude psychopharmacological interventions. The child learns. Synaptic connections are made and broken. Fear and joy involve the activation of huge neural nets which in turn drive physiological hormone release, heart rate, and immune functions. We can manipulate some of these systems with pharmacological tools acting on monoaminergic pathways or we can manipulate them by good and bad news acting selectively through those same pathways. By mechanisms we do not yet understand, the firing of some neurons creates, in the optic cortex, the color green, which somehow, magically, we perceive. The firing of others creates sensations we call pain, while the action potentials of still others produce sensations we call pleasure. How these well-defined firing patterns create these sensations is not clear. Nor is it clear how such diverse sensations as sex and the taste of chocolate ice cream are lumped together as pleasurable, while the sharpness of a toothache and the dull ache of the intestine are somehow universally classified as pain. Both are susceptible to endogenous as well exogenous chemical intervention. One can adapt to some pains. One can be bored by some pleasures.

Neurobiology has clearly demonstrated central effects on the immune system, on hormonal balance, and on blood flow, many of which are under direct control of the conscious mind. Again, we know that people can be scared to death, that the placebo effect is real, and that the will to live can alter clinical course. What we do not know is how to use these responses effectively. Yet, conversation, social support, and tender loving care are important therapeutic tools, although, as Freud noted, they are mostly effective in the medical treatment of relatively mild neurotic states. Indeed, it was their ineffectiveness in psychosis that led to the rise of psychopharmacology.

The great problem in medicine is always evaluation, and the problem is especially difficult in evaluating psychotherapy and psychodynamic procedures. Whether Freudian, Jungian, Adlerian, Rogerian, Gestalt, Existential, Skinarian, Pavlovian, or whatever, the goal is to gain control of the unconscious sources of motivation in the belief that such access will alleviate the clinical problem. But how to assess efficacy and identify appropriate target populations is still obscure. That some psychotherapeutic procedures are helpful to some individuals is clearly the case, but the issues of what is effective and for whom are unclear. No two psychotherapists function in the same way even when trained in the same school, nor are any two patients alike. Rather, each psychotherapist is like a violinist who uniquely renders a composer's work to thrill some members of the audience but bore others. To carry the analogy further, like music, the timing and content of therapeutic interventions are critical to the therapeutic response, and each therapist is idiosyncratically sensitive to particular situations. "To have said a thing before its time is never to have said it at all," and to say a thing at the wrong time may cause considerable emotional distress, just as the timing and content of words can lead to a marriage or to its dissolution. As a result, despite a voluminous literature, psychotherapy is still much more an art than a science, and the results are no less difficult to quantify. This does not mean that such therapy cannot or should not be quantified but rather that insufficient work has been carried out yet to do so. It is much needed.

2.3 General methods

2.3.1 Behavioral methods

2.3.1.1 Clinical observations

Psychiatric research is concerned both with the brain and its manifestation, the mind. Accordingly, it encompasses both biology and behavior, for the two are clearly linked. Indeed, it is this linkage that makes psychiatry in particular so difficult because the mind is as much an activity of the brain as insulin is a product of pancreatic beta cells. It is this linkage between the organ and its manifestation that we regard as "us" that we find so terrifying. We would like to believe that somehow our mind is independent of the organ. Yet, psychiatric syndromes such as depression and schizophrenia, neurological ones such as Alzheimer's and Huntington's, and the clear mental changes induced by the physical trauma of strokes, brain damage, and psychoactive drugs show us how weak that belief is — and that threatens our conception of ourselves.

Close clinical observation and accurate descriptions of the character and course of disease are important areas of research, and there is plenty of room in science for case studies. Indeed, nearly every disease and syndrome in medicine was first identified in a careful case study and only later verified in larger, more controlled studies. There is currently no substitute for the human mind and the clinician's careful eye which distinguish the features of a single individual from those around him. On the one hand, case studies are the initiating process in medical science, raising questions and developing hypotheses for study. On the other, it is the least reliable procedure for verification and assessing significance. While disease identification and the discovery of idiosyncratic responses to the environment or to therapies are vital to medicine, once they have been detected larger clinical studies are required to verify the incidence and significance of what was identified. And, to the extent that case studies are qualitative rather then quantitative, there is little that can be said here beyond such homilies as "look carefully." Though the brain and behavior are linked, for ease of discussion they are discussed separately below.

2.3.1.2 Rating scales

Rating scales are the most commonly used instruments in psychiatric research. Their primary purposes are to objectify and quantify behavioral observations and to permit statistical comparisons of changes within and between populations. Despite their use and number, much of the rich complexity of human behavior is not easily quantified. Qualitative observations and assessments are still needed for their own sake as well as to identify areas requiring more quantitative evaluation. Nor are rating scales the only possible tools for objectifying behavior, as will be discussed later. Despite these limitations, rating scales are enormously useful and are the backbone of much psychiatric research.

2.3.1.2.1 Types. Three major kinds of rating scales have been developed. Some quantify general morbidity, such as the Iowa Structured Psychiatric Interview (SPI), which is intended for epidemiological survey of populations for psychiatric disease. Others are intended to objectify diagnosis. One example is the Structured Clinical Interview for the DSM-n (SCID; DSM-n is the acronym for the *Diagnostic and Statistical Manual of Mental Disorders*, developed by the American Psychiatric Association to operationally define psychiatric diagnosis). Another commonly used scale for this purpose is the Brief Psychiatric Rating Scale (BPRS). Finally, there are scales to objectify changes in the symptom severity. An example is the Hamilton Depression Scale (HRSD).

Obviously, just as one would not use a saw to do the work of a wrench, so it is important that rating scales be chosen with careful consideration of their suitability to the task. Scales designed for one purpose may or may not be applicable for another. The IQ test, for example, was designed to predict scholastic achievement and should not be assumed to identify "intelligence," even though scholastic achievement may require some level of some kinds of intelligence. Not only does the IQ test measure other traits as well, but intelligence itself is also a very broad series of traits, not all of which are applicable to acquiring scholastic skills. In a similar fashion, a test designed to measure depression may not be suitable to measure "negative symptoms," although some "negative symptoms" may be related to underlying depression.

The form of the data to be used should also be considered. The most powerful data for statistical treatment are parametric data. These are continuous real numbers that have a real zero and continuous intervals between values. Examples would be height and weight, which, even though limited to a small range of all possible values, nonetheless consist of real numbers and continuous intervals.

Ordinal data, like parametric data, are real numbers with a real zero, but they are discontinuous. Heart rate is one example.

There either is, or is not, a measured heartbeat, and there is a constant numeric interval between the numbers even though in some forms of heart disease the temporal interval between heartbeats is not. Similarly, the number of offspring is also a whole number with a constant numeric interval between them, regardless of differences in age or personality. Most data in clinical studies, however, have neither a true zero nor constant intervals between numbers. Instead, the numbers are crudely representative of relationships. Scalar data are comparative and include such things as changes in clinical state, severity, or some other subjective or psychological response. Such rankings are generally not quantitative but rather global and are often characterized by preceding adjectives such as "better," "worse," slightly," very," etc. The intervals between such rankings are seldom uniform and the rankings themselves are not uniformly continuous.

Another common kind of data is ordinal, with a general ranking and a zero but generally without uniform intervals between rankings. These data include items such as severity. Here the modifiers are generally the adjectives "more" and "less." Finally, there are categorical data, which divide data into classes such as diagnosis, gender, education, ethnicity, etc.

The ease of extracting meaning from a rating scale depends a good deal on how well the numbers can be made to fit the basic assumptions of statistical manipulation. Generally, the more parametric, the easier the analysis. An additional factor is the clarity of the ratings, and these are generally best when specific reference points are included.

Who is going to do the rating should also be considered. Some scales are intended for self-administration. Some can be carried out by ward personnel other than a psychiatrist. Still others require a trained psychiatrist. Who is required depends both on the nature of the study and the available facilities.

Two critical features of any scale are its validity and its reliability. These are not the same. It is possible to have great validity and poor reliability or great reliability of a totally invalid scale. Validity refers to accuracy in measuring that which the scale is intended to measure. It is, to use a common example in statistical texts, the bull's eye of a target. Simply because a scale is named, for example, the "Smerdloo Anxiety Test," does not necessarily mean it really does measure "anxiety." Its validity has to be established. Similarly, even if the test is valid, it may be so difficult to administer or so subject to bias and change that the results are unreliable. It is like knowing where the bull's eye is on the target but being unable to shoot that far away with any accuracy. Reliability, therefore, like validity, needs to be established for any rating scale.

2.3.1.2.2 Validity. Validity can be established directly or indirectly. Direct or "face validity" exists when what is to be measured is directly related to the measure. This is the case, for example, if playing the violin is used to measure the ability to play the violin. If etiology is known, validity can be assessed by correspondence with the etiology. This has been termed "criterion validity." Unfortunately, in psychiatry, most syndromes are essentially mental constructs of unknown etiology. There is, therefore, no "true" known etiological agent against which to assess the validity of a test; rather, one is forced to rely upon concordance with scales intended to measure the essential features of the mental construct. Appropriately enough, this is named "construct validity." For example, one might wish to measure the construct "honesty" by developing questions assessing the limits for honest responses. Later scales might then take their correspondence with this scale as a measure of their own validity.

Obviously, this kind of bootstrap assessment is only as good as whatever is taken as the standard and is really an exercise in circular reasoning. However, the strength of an association with a construct can be increased by measures that differ in kind. Correlating a behavioral "anxiety" scale with a physiological measure of "anxiety" (e.g., the galvanic skin response), an endocrinological measure of "anxiety" (e.g., glucorticoid elevations), and a metabolic measure of anxiety (e.g., increased norepinephrine release around blood vessels) is more convincing than correlating it with a dozen other behavioral scales dependent on the true validity of some primary behavioral scale.

The predictive value of a test also lends it credence. The IQ test was created to predict academic performance. Its validity depends upon its ability to do so. A rating scale measuring anxiety should similarly reflect subjective anxiety.

The major difficulty in testing the validity of rating scales, then, is in operationally defining the primary referent even though its general definition is taken to be clear. As someone once said about stress studies, "...The most stressful thing in defining stress is that everyone understands what the word means but they differ in their understanding." So, too, with many terms for symptomatic states. Everyone knows what they mean, but to each the meaning is idiosyncratic. One function of rating scales, whatever their intrinsic validity, is to provide an operational definition to a primary referent. A diagnostic rating scale such as the DSM-n provides operational definitions of syndromes whose real validity may not necessarily be accepted by all and may not, in fact, point to underlying etiologies. Indeed, the fact that it is the DSM-n, where "n" is whatever revision is in current use, rather than DMS-I, II, III, IV, or IVR, attests to the conflicts and difficulties in operationally defining some of the constructs. The more specifically defined the terms, however, the easier it is to devise valid means for their measurement.

2.3.1.2.3 Reliability. It is much easier to determine if everyone is marching in step than if they are going in the right direction. So, too, is it easier to assess reliability than validity. The reliability of a test procedure is an empirical measure of concordance between raters. It is different than the reliability of responses by the subject.

Two measures are of importance in assessing reliability. First is the consistency of an observer's ratings over time; this is "test-retest" reliability. Second is the constancy of rating between individuals, or inter-rater reliability. Both drift. Extreme values generally tend to diminish with experience and time as still more extreme instances occur. Similarly, because individuals differ in experience and learning, inter-rater reliability may also begin to drift.

To guard against drift and to obtain consistent concordance between raters, a period of initial training is generally required to clarify the operational meaning of terms and the scoring procedures and criteria. Repetitive ratings of videotapes or re-evaluations of the same population over time can be used to detect and correct observer drift. In principle, the interval between reassessments should be short enough to minimize drift and changes in the population but long enough to minimize reflexive ratings. As always, the more specific and operationally defined the terms in a rating scale, the easier it is to achieve and maintain reliability. Thus, it is easier to get agreement on something such as the distance between two objects than on something such as the "quality of life." This is also true for the subject when self-rating tests are used. In this instance, confusion in the terms will lead to inconsistent responses, and often rating forms are devised to access the same information in more than one way in order to assess the reliability of self-rated measures. Also, alternative forms of the rating may be prepared and administered at different times and in different order to prevent learning effects.

Establishing validity and reliability takes a major effort, so careful consideration should be given to using existing accepted scales before deciding to develop a new one. The use of established scales has the added advantage of simplifying comparison with the existing literature. Results obtained with idiosyncratic scales sometimes linger outside the mainstream until the scale items are assessed and accepted. Of course, sometimes existing scales are inadequate for a particular task and a new one must be devised. Like all methods development, however, establishing validity and reliability may become a research project within the research project.

Although plentiful, scales vary considerably in personnel requirements, what the ratings cover, the time required for their completion, the kinds of data produced, and whether the scales are administered in a free or structured setting. Any of these factors may influence the suitability of a particular scale at specific sites. Almost all diagnostic rating schedules require physicians or trained personnel; therefore, they are somewhat expensive to administer. On the other hand, some of the scales assessing general morbidity or changes in symptoms are self-administered and somewhat less expensive. However, their use predicates both competence and motivation on the part of the rater in order to provide an honest and accurate assessment. Not all subjects possess either. The number of items and the time for completion are also of practical importance. In self-administered tests, motivation often declines with effort; the greater the number of items, the less motivated the rater may be to complete them. If clinicians or trained personnel are required, the cost of their time goes up with the number of items that require evaluation.

A listing of many of the existing rating scales and a brief discussion of their features can be found in chapters by Dennis (1992), Murphy (1992), and Tyrer (1992). A more complete reference and evaluation list, continually updated by the World Health Organization, can be found at the web site:

www.who.int/msa/cidi/literature.htm

2.3.1.3 *Other behavioral measures*

While of undeniable utility, rating scales are not the only way to quantify behavior or even necessarily the best method, although they are certainly among the most convenient. As indicated above, rating scales are an attempt to objectify emotional and behavioral status by pen-and-pencil questionnaires. Most of us, however, continually monitor the emotional and behavioral status of those around us by nearly automatically observing and recording subtle, quantifiable nonverbal changes in posture, expression, and even gait. Every artist and cartoonist depends on such observations. A small shift in eyebrows, a turn of the mouth, a tightening of an eyelid … all convey information. The phrases "they were very close" or "we have drifted apart" are merely verbal reflections of subtle differences in standing distance accompanying such emotional relationships. A couple invades each other's standing space in intimate conversation, while antagonists stand apart. Cultural differences in such customs even have international consequences. Scandinavians are thought cold because of the greater distance between them in casual conversation as compared to that of Americans, while Italians seem warm because they stand closer. Individuals in all cultures, however, are equally passionate and equally aloof.

The manner of walking conveys information. The strut is not the droop. Walking "the wrong way" can invite attack in some areas of a city but be a social grace in others. Indeed, everyone has had the experience of entering into a room full of strangers and knowing almost instantly who will accept and who will reject social interactions. Sometimes these assumptions are in error, but more often they are not.

It is these nonverbal responses that permit the study of behavior in prevocal periods of human infancy and are used to quantify animal behavior. Their occurrence, frequency, and duration reveal much about the emotional and cognitive status of the subjects. Some of these factors have also been applied in clinical settings as well, although not as often as they might. Among the fully quantitative measures which have been or which could be used in assessing behavior and behavioral changes are such things as standing distance between subjects and between subjects and ward personnel, eye-blink rate in response to questions, postural changes, sleep duration and sleep onset, activity level, saccadic movements, changes in the angle of the eyelid and the corners of the mouth, etc. All afford quantifiable or potentially quantifiable measures of behavior that can be scored directly in focal sessions or from videotapes to avoid observer influences over the variables of interest. This is an important area for future research that is held back largely by an unawareness of the richness of such observations, by the speeds at which they occur, and by the time required for training and in making the observations themselves. Development in this area should increase with the technical advances being made in image capture and analysis.

2.3.2   *Biological measures*

A plenitude of biological measures is currently available to medicine and psychiatry and more measures are added daily. No attempt can be made in this small handbook to discuss or even enumerate them all in detail. Rather, this section is limited to some general considerations of principles and caveats.

2.3.2.1   *Physiological measures*

To the many new measures added to such standard physiological variables as heart rate, blood pressure, skin conductance, diagnostic EEGs, and the like have now been added the imaging marvels of CT, MRI, PET, SPECT, and ERP-power-spectra and newer immunoassays for hormones, cytokines, and cell markers. These, together with rapid advances in the neurosciences in general, have enormously impacted psychiatric research. For the first time, it is possible to examine the static and functional human brain and the immunological and endocrine cascades accompanying mental disease. The former possibility has led to a great resurgence in attempts to relate anatomical alterations to disease, the latter to an extended examination of the role of "stress" in human disease.

2.3.2.1.1 Imaging. The two complementary techniques, computerized tomography (CT) and magnetic resonance imaging (MRI), allow for a detailed anatomical examination in living creatures. Three others — functional MRI (fMRI), positron emission tomography (PET), and single photon emission computed tomography (SPECT) — provide some information on metabolism, while event-related potentials (ERP) give a detailed view of ongoing neural activity. Based on separate principles, the techniques in combination can roughly locate not only the anatomy of many neural events but also some of the accompanying physiological and biochemical concomitants. In addition, rapid advances in technology are quickly overcoming the limitations of the various methods and increasing their strengths.

Computerized tomography, like classical X-ray, images by measuring tissue density. Dense tissues, such as bone, absorb more X-ray energy than do softer tissues. CT differs in that it uses a rotating array of detectors, thereby providing a three-dimensional image of the tissue.

In contrast to CT, MRI images more indirectly by assessing the density and orientation in tissue of paramagnetic materials, primarily the protons in water, but it can detect other materials as well (see discussion on MRS below). Unlike X-rays, the image is not affected by bone calcium or other dense materials which do not have unpaired electrons. Because both proton density, but especially viscosity, and the electric fields of adjacent molecules vary between tissues, the technique allows for great detail. Basically, it consists of aligning the protons in tissue in a magnetic field, perturbing that orientation with a specific radiofrequency pulse (the Lamar frequency), and measuring the rate of return to the prestimulus condition upon termination of the pulse. Two major properties are measured: the rate of return to the orientation of the magnetic field and the dephasing of the magnetic moment. The first is measured as T1 and is called the spin-lattice relaxation time, while the second is referred to as T2, the spin-

spin relaxation time. T1, technically, is defined as the time required to reduce the difference between the longitudinal magnetic field and its equilibrium value to *e*. T2 is the time required to reduce transverse magnetization by a factor of *e*. T1 and T2 are differentially sensitive to density, viscosity, and adjacent materials, and each records different intensities of signal from different tissues. As a result, a variety of timing and intensity protocols is available to weight signals toward T1 or T2, depending upon diagnostic need.

A modification of the standard procedure can be also be used to estimate local blood flow. Functional MRI (fMRI) derives from the observation that oxyhemoglobin and dexohemoglobin differ in their magnetic properties and can be imaged using the proper settings, so-called BOD (blood oxygen dependent) settings. By taking advantage of this property, along with faster imaging techniques and growing information on the linkage between cerebrovascular blood flow and neural activity, fMRI has been used to examine regional brain activity during neural events by recording changes in blood flow. This is sometimes referred to as an event-related MRI.

Magnetic resonance spectroscopy (MRS) has even greater potential. By judicious selection of protocols, *in situ* semi-quantitative estimates of a variety of endogenous metabolites can be made. These include neuronal markers such as *N*-acetylaspartate, glial markers such as myoinositol, membrane markers such as choline, nitrate and nitrite marking NO regulation, and energy metabolites such as glucose, lactate, pyruvate, and creatine-creatine phosphate. The list grows daily. In addition, the procedure allows tracking of fluoro-derivates of pharmacological agents. Although the power of MRS is in its infancy, it has already made substantive contributions to the diagnosis and treatment of neurological diseases and of metabolic errors in neonates. Although it has yet to prove its worth in psychiatry, it is a very potent tool for psychiatric studies.

Among other things, PET can be used to estimate local metabolic response to stimuli. The procedure is based on the principle that the nuclear decay of some isotopes produces a positron which immediately combines with an electron. The resultant annihilation energy emerges at right angles from the annihilation site as a pair of high-energy (511-KeV) photons.

These can be detected and their source determined. The most commonly used isotopes are C-11 (half-life, 20 min), N-13 (half-life, 10 min), and O-15 (half-life, 2 min), as these elements are the stuff of life. Fl-18 (half-life, 110 min) is also very commonly used in the form of fluoro-derivatives of biological materials of interest. Because of the very short half-lives of these isotopes, large doses of radioactivity can be used with minimal radiation exposure. However, the short half-lives also require almost *in situ* synthesis of the test compounds. Indeed, most facilities using PET have their own cyclotron to produce the isotopes and a team of organic chemists to rapidly synthesize the compounds to be used. The cost, then, is considerable, and the compounds are limited to those that can be prepared rapidly and with great purity.

Despite these drawbacks, PET is an enormously useful technique with broad applications. One important use is to estimate local glucose metabolism. This procedure is based on the observation that 2-deoxyglucose is transported into cells on the glucose carrier at nearly the same rate as glucose itself. Once in the cell, the 2-deoxyglucose cannot be further catabolized. Fl-18-2-deoxyglucose acts like 2-deoxyglucose and can be used to measure its regional uptake. This can then be matched with blood flow measured by PET, using O-15 containing water or butanol, or with the blood flow changes detected with event-related MRI. At the other extreme, fluoro-analogues of receptor agonists and antagonists permit rough measures of regional receptor density. Not only are PET applications to the neurosciences extensive, but they are also perhaps even more valuable to clinical oncology and cardiology.

Single photon emission computed tomography suffers from being less quantitative and less anatomically specific than PET but is considerably less expensive and, if combined with MRI, can provide much useful information. In contrast to PET, the radiolabeled agents used in SPECT emit only a single high-energy photon. While the two photons in PET, because they are emitted at right angles from their point of origin, allow for exact localization, the absorption and scatter of the single photon from SPECT radionucleides complicate localization and quantitation. The major use of SPECT in neurobiology is to evaluate regional blood flow with technetium-99 (140-KeV photon, 6-hr half-life), usually bound to hexamethylpropylamine oxime (Tc-99-HMPAO), with iodine-123 (159-KeV photon; 12-hr half-life) incorporated into I-123-isopropyliodoamphetamine or, much less commonly, xenon-133 (80-KeV photon; 5.3-day half-life) administered by breathing. Iodine derivatives of agonists and antagonists have also been used to image receptor binding sites. In some studies, the quantitation, after appropriate corrections for emitter absorption by tissue, is nearly as good as that obtained using PET.

These techniques have raised important new questions about the physiology of the brain. As examples, glucose consumption as measured in these studies exceeds oxygen supply and is not necessarily commensurate with neural firing rate. The linkages thus require clarification, as does the considerable time lag between the institution of neural activity and increased blood flow. While changes in blood flow are generally related to the complexity of the task, the circulatory system is a closed loop and increased flow in one area requires a decrease elsewhere. While today's emphasis is on the increase in flow, the decrease, though more difficult to detect, will also become of interest. Coupling the changes in blood flow with alterations in metabolite concentrations as detected by MRS should vastly increase our understanding of the neural substrate to some behaviors.

While the temporal resolution of all these methods improves daily, regional blood flow, glucose metabolism, and changes in metabolite production, whatever their final correlation with neural activity and with each other, are still hundreds of milliseconds slower than the neural events they seek to examine. On the other hand, multichannel ERP taken from scalp electrodes can more closely track regional neural events in real time but at the cost of some uncertainty as to the origin of the signals, the so-called "inverse problem." Basically, ERP consists of wedding the field potentials of classical multichannel EEG with fast computer transforms. The result is a continual picture of neural activity at selected frequencies. Combining this with neuroimaging of blood flow, glucose uptake, ligand binding, or metabolite distribution embeds the temporal activity into a spatial matrix.

In addition to the electrical phenomena accompanying the ion flows that make for neural firing are magnetic phenomena, as well. While these are exceedingly weak, much current work is dedicated to assessing their utility.

The great value of these methodologies, especially in concert, to tracking the anatomy and circuitry of many behavioral responses is obvious. The major problems are in defining the initiating events; that is, in identifying the neural source of volition and in deciphering the significance of the neural events. In one sense, the current status of imaging is comparable to locating the factory carrying out an operation. However, somewhere between the alerting signal (and, in some cases, perhaps even before it), a decision must be made in response to the alerting signal. The neurons involved in making that decision may be too few in number to be assessed right now. It is those neurons, however, that are critical in the operation, just as directions from the executive office are critical to operations on the assembly line.

The second problem, as once stated by Kety, is that it probably takes as much energy to think a stupid thought as a smart one. The methods we have discussed here show neural activity, but whether that activity is inhibitory or stimulatory, productive or unproductive, creative or repetitive cannot yet be determined, at least by these methods. Clearly, this is an area that requires considerable more work, although combining MRI spectroscopy with the other techniques will at least provide a real-time image of the biochemical and electrical events in the neural factory involved in a particular behavioral change. Much of this is yet to come.

2.3.2.1.2 Endocrine cascades. A second area of great advances in medical physiology is that of neuroendocrinology. Again, there can be no attempt here to cover this vast area in any detail. Increasingly, however, the steps and mechanisms between neural control of hormonal release and their feedback interactions have been clarified over the years.

Although it is abundantly clear that many hormones, perhaps all, affect human behavior, psychiatry has largely concentrated on gonadal hormones and the stress response. Interest in the former is often attributed to Freud, although interest in sex certainly predates him. Indeed, randomization of the gene pool is of such biological utility that, to look at it coldly, an elaborate set of behaviors has evolved to assure its continuation, and much of our lives is governed by the emotional attachments driven by the presence or absence of testosterone on the hypothalamus at critical periods in development. Detailing those periods and defining the mechanisms involved in human sexuality are important areas of neurobiology research and, ultimately, clinical psychiatry. Yet, despite the development of direct medical treatments for some forms of sexual malfunction, there are no effective biological treatments yet for the emotional problems stemming from sexual desire and rejection. Psychotherapy, in one form or another, is still required to treat such problems.

Psychiatric interest in "stressors" and the "stress response" derives from animal and human studies showing physiological and behavioral consequences of exposure to "stressors." This, together with some clinical observations, has led to the belief that social stressors may precipitate some of the major psychiatric illnesses including schizophrenia and bipolar depression. In support, most studies show that concordance for clinical schizophrenia or bipolar disorder among identical twins is not absolute but rather occurs in a range between 40 and 60% in various studies, regardless of whether the twins are raised together or separately. Indeed, this figure seems to be typical for most, if not all, major psychiatric disorders. This is taken to indicate that genetics alone is not sufficient to account for disease manifestation and that the remainder is due to some unspecified stressors. Much work has been devoted to identifying those stressors within the family or society in the hope that they may be more amenable to therapeutic manipulation than genetics. Of course, gene expression itself is modifiable by environmental factors, and genetic manipulation, with all its philosophical and ethical problems, is becoming increasingly possible. And, of course, gene interactions could also account for the variable occurrence of symptoms if these syndromes were under only multigenetic control.

The stress response has also been of interest as a possible predictor of disease vulnerability, onset, clinical course, or response to treatment. The seeming increase in the occurrence of mood swings, depression, and suicide in the population and the growing number of "stressors" in everyday life have also helped stimulate interest in the stress response.

Difficulties in interpreting many "stress" studies, however, include clearly specifying stress procedures, defining "stress" itself, and examining the data without regard to the evolutionary function of the stress response. That is, many experimental paradigms, especially in animals, use as stressors conditions which, despite their ease of replication and ability to activate the pituitary-adrenal axis, are never encountered in nature so that the consequent responses are often difficult to interpret in biological terms. For example, while response to an electrical grid is easily quantified in animal studies, such electric shocks to the feet are never encountered in nature and response to them is by translation to something else.

A stressor, in the broad sense, is anything that upsets metabolic equilibrium and calls for readjustment to homeostasis. Physiologically, stressors are defined by activation of the hypothalamic-pituitary-adrenal axis. The real stressors faced by animals in the wild, and by all humans before "civilization" some 10,000 years ago, were thirst, hunger, heat, cold, infection, and tissue damage.

Correspondingly, stress responses evolved over the course of evolution to shape behavior and metabolism to overcome these disruptions and return to the basal state. Early studies showed that these stressors elicited stress-specific patterns of hormone release. Many of the metabolic mechanisms elicited by these hormones were defined during the period when biochemical research was directed toward elucidating intermediary metabolism. Although less was done to examine the metabolic consequences of the hormonal interactions occurring after real stressors, a general picture emerged that these hormones were released in a stressor-specific time and magnitude-dependent manner to permit metabolic adaptations that restore physiological balance.

Perhaps the most heavily studied of the hormonal responses to stress is the major marker for stress itself, activation of the hypothalamic-pituitary-adrenal axis. Such activation is the physiological equivalent of the permissive beat, common to all music, while other hormones play the metabolic tunes specific to each stressors.

Evolution shapes both biology and behavior, for the two are inexorably linked. This linkage is especially evident in the endocrine cascade of the stress response which not only controls metabolic adaptations, but behavior as well. Thus, corticotrophin-releasing factor (CRF) released from the preoptic area of the hypothalamus within seconds of a stimulus such as tissue damage increases arousal and decreases feeding behavior, as does adrenocorticotropic hormone (ACTH) released from the pituitary which also sharpens memory. These are critical to the animal's survival. The physiological function of ACTH is to release glucocorticoids from the adrenal, and glucocorticoids hasten forgetting and blunt memory, which, again, is critical if animals are to avoid living in constant terror. Metabolically, glucocorticoids start a cascade of enzymatic inductions, largely geared toward decreasing protein synthesis and increasing the conversion of amino acids to glucose. Some of these are repressed, however, if glucose is already present in sufficient quantities to sustain increased metabolism or if other specific hormones, such as growth hormone, are concomitantly released.

The cascade of glucocorticoid-driven enzyme inductions depends on the persistence and magnitude of the stressor. For example, ornithine decarboxylase activity is increased within minutes of corticoid administration; tyrosine transaminase and tryptophan pyrrolase, within 5 hr; and alanine transaminase, in 24 hr. It should be noted, however, that while some hormones such as glucocorticoids directly induce metabolic enzymes, others regulate metabolic activity by such mechanisms as stimulating kinases to carry out metabolic commands. In nearly all cases, however, the end result is to promote physiological recovery. And, as with the hormonal changes eliciting glucocorticoid release, the metabolic changes induced by other stress hormones also affect behavior. Again, body and brain are a single biological unit and the effects of peripheral metabolism on the brain and behavior are no less important or profound than those of the neural activity on peripheral metabolism. An example of this is the effect of glucocorticoids and other hormones on tryptophan metabolism and its consequences for the status of the central transmitter serotonin. This linkage depends on the substrate dependency of the rate-limiting step in serotonin biosynthesis, tryptophan hydroxylase. This is an unusual phenomenon. Most branch-point enzymes are enzyme limited and subject to endpoint feedback. A second part of the linkage to behavior results from the fact that tryptophan is transported into the brain on a neutral amino acid carrier and so must compete with other neutral amino acids such as phenylalanine, tyrosine, leucine, etc. for passage.

Stressors, then, affect peripheral tryptophan in three ways. First, the stress-induced release of norepinephrine and epinephrine from the adrenal medulla increases fatty acid release. These fatty acids, in turn, displace tryptophan from the albumin binding sites necessary to transport this relatively insoluble compound. Fatty acid occupation of these sites then increases the free-to-bound tryptophan ratio. If the stressor continues long enough, and glucose levels do not repress induction, elevated corticoids eventually induce the activities of tryptophan transaminase and hepatic tryptophan pyrrolase. Tryptophan transaminase removes tryptophan by converting it to indolepyruvic acid. Quantitatively much more important, tryptophan pyrrolase splits the indole ring irrevocably, committing tryptophan to catabolism. On this degradative pathway, tryptophan catabolites form the inhibitor of glutamate receptors, kynurenic acid, and the N-methyl-d-aspartate (NMDA) receptor agonist, quinolinic acid, as well as nicotinic acid (a similar sequence of reactions is carried out in brain, mediated by tryptophan-2-3-deoxygenase, which is induced, not by corticoids, but by interferon). If insulin is also released, so are the neutral amino acids which compete with tryptophan for passage through the blood-brain barrier. Concomitantly, protein synthesis is slowed, as not only is tryptophan one of the limiting essential amino acids in protein synthesis but it also helps stabilize polysomes. The end consequence of all this enormously simplified litany is that blood tryptophan concentration is reduced under some conditions of stress, thereby reducing brain serotonin, increasing unease, and stimulating searching activity.

Intricate as these metabolic dances may be, the problem for psychiatry is that the stressors of civilization generally have no metabolic answer. The demands of work or home are products of our civilization, and 10,000 years is insufficient time to have developed appropriate biological responses to these stressors, even if there were some evolutionary mechanism selecting for their development. As a consequence, the body struggles to maintain an emotional equilibrium which is unattainable by metabolic means. Weight loss is common as the body tries one metabolic approach, or weight gain as it tries another. Sleep is disturbed, and unease common. The literature indicates that chronic unremitting corticoid elevations in response to stressors reduces the number of killer T-cells and thus immunological potency; if such a pattern is chronically sustained, it may even lead to the glutamate-driven death of hippocampal and other neurons. It is not a matter, then, of the stress response evolving to kill us but rather that we have, in our short time on Earth, changed what the response needs to do to help us survive. While clinicians cannot change the sources of stress, they can identify them and assist subjects by behavioral or pharmacological means to oppose their evolutionary response to stressors, with all its immunological and neural consequences.

2.3.2.2 *Biochemical measures*

The mind is related to the activity of the brain in much the same way as albumin is related to liver function. Imaging techniques, especially PET and SPECT, are approaches to obtaining anatomical and some relatively gross biochemical information on the living brain. Most of the search for biochemical concomitants of disease, however, are carried out on dead tissue, cells, or tissue in culture; on the constituents of one of the body's fluids: blood, urine, saliva, or cerebrospinal fluid; or on animals. Each of these systems provides different information.

Even more diverse are biochemical methodologies and approaches. On the one hand is the systems approach, weaving biochemical strands into the rope of life. On the other is the examination of the structure of the strands themselves, a journey from physiological biochemistry to chemical biochemistry to biochemical genetics. It would be impossible here to even attempt to recount the status of today's understanding of neurobiology, which expands daily. Instead, this section is limited to some general comments about the tissues available for study and the areas of major concern to psychiatric biochemical research today, transmitter systems, receptors, and the cascade of secondary and tertiary messengers.

2.3.2.2.1 Tissues: **Brain autopsy material.** New histochemical and molecular biological techniques have made possible examination of the detailed chemistry of the autopsied brain in the same way that advances in selective staining allowed detailed examination of its anatomy. Moreover, using immunological procedures, the same piece of tissue can be successively examined for many receptors and metabolites, providing a fantastic wealth of detailed information on the *in situ* biochemistry of the brain. As a consequence, there is growing use of normal and pathological brain tissue in the search for understanding normal brain function as well as disease etiology, and tissue banks will now supply qualified investigators with carefully defined autopsy material.

There are, of course, problems in looking at autopsied material. If life is a steady-state equilibrium removed from thermodynamic equilibrium, then death is thermodynamic equilibrium and dead tissue eventually reaches that lowest thermodynamic state. Fortunately, not all systems get there immediately, and, the changes are very slow for some systems. Just as most of what we know about neurochemistry comes from fresh animal tissue, human tissue can be equally informative, depending on pre- and postmortem treatments. Thus, the concentrations of acetylcholine or gamma-aminobutyric acid (GABA) in autopsied brain likely bear no relationship to the concentrations in living brain. On the other hand, the concentrations of gangliosides, many enzymes, and many structural proteins may. The status of still others, such as some receptors and some specific enzymes, may reflect premortem and agonal events, as well. Caution is required, for example, in interpreting population differences in receptor numbers in a disease where disease treatment itself influences receptor number. That is, as in everything else, care is required in selecting the variables to be studied and in interpreting the findings. Care is also necessary when deciding where to look. The brain is enormous at the level of histochemistry and enormously compartmentalized and complex at any level.

Other tissues. Whatever is found in dead brain is of little value to its owner. Other tissues are needed to find biological markers of disease etiology or predictors of treatment which are immediately applicable to the living. Among the tissue so studied are patient-derived cells in tissue culture. Skin fibroblasts and immortalized lymphocytes are among the easiest to obtain. Both are used as a source of genomic DNA for linkage studies aimed at detecting genetic contributions to disease state, and both have been used to examine for genetic control of particular biochemical systems. For example, fibroblasts contain monoamine oxidase A (MAO-A), the major enzyme in monoamine metabolism, and there are significant differences in the MAO activity of different fibroblast lines. Similarly, lymphocytes contain beta-adrenergic receptors and can be used to examine factors affecting receptor regulation. Better and better techniques have been developed for studying specific cell types such as glia, and neurons in pure or mixed cultures have permitted direct measures of cellular interactions, sources for the factors responsible for such interactions, the mechanisms of action of growth factors, and nearly all aspects of cellular neurobiology. The caveat, of course, is that such cells are free of the normal constraints and regulations seen within a tissue, and what is observed is the range of potential responses and not necessarily those occurring *in situ*.

Blood. Blood is probably the most common source of biochemical information used in medicine, and the blood stream has been likened to a red highway carrying supplies to far-flung cells. Like a highway, it contains organelles, and, like a highway, its composition may vary from time to time in accordance with tissue needs. As a result, a blood sample drawn at a particular time provides information on blood composition at the moment it was drawn. The concentrations of many blood components are well regulated and for them variations are small. Others, however, such as melatonin, adrenal hormones, and pituitary hormones, undergo marked circadian variations, and timing becomes critical to interpretation.

The major organelles in blood are also potential sources of information. Particular interest has focused on properties that may be analogous to those in the central nervous system or may be of value in diagnosing metabolic errors. Thus, among a host of other metabolic systems, erythrocytes contain catechol-O-methyltransferase, one of the enzymes of catecholamine catabolism, and porphobilinogen deaminase, which is of importance in diagnosing porphyria. Platelets contain serotonin storage vesicles, a serotonin re-uptake system, 5HT2 receptors linked to shape change, an alpha2-adrenergic receptor, and monoamine oxidase B. Leukocytes have beta-adrenergic receptors. Further, the organelles in the blood of different species may provide a source for other variables of interest. For example, while human platelets contain MAO-B, those of other species contain MAO-A.

Saliva. Phlebotomy is traumatic to many individuals, but the discovery that the concentration of many pharmacologic agents in saliva is in equilibrium with that in blood has made saliva a viable alternative in some studies. The greatest difficulty is in collecting a sufficient sample. Stimulation of saliva production by chewing on wax is a common procedure.

Urine. While blood provides a look at the instantaneous flow of materials between tissues, urine is the dump site for most of the products and catabolites consumed or produced by the body during the interval between collections. However, just as a midden provides a clever archeologist with the information needed to reconstruct a civilization, so can urine provide information necessary to reconstruct the metabolic status of the host. Care should be taken, however, to make sure that drug and dietary components in the urine are not mistaken for metabolic abnormality in the experimental population.

Cerebrospinal fluid. Cerebrospinal fluid (CSF) is essentially a partial urine of the brain and, like urine from the periphery, is of considerable value in examining the status of brain and spinal cord biochemistry. Many of the metabolites appearing in CSF are also more directly transported out of brain into the blood. Of course, like urine, CSF provides a global status devoid of anatomical specificity, and it is important to recognize the contributions of the cord, especially when examining for metabolites that occur in both tissues. Because spinal fluid is a standing column of liquid, concentration gradients may exist for some compounds depending on their anatomical origin. For example, heavy contributions from the brain must diffuse to lumbar sites, and the concentrations of these materials vary with volume in passive collection. This is the case, for example, with many monoamine metabolites.

Nevertheless, the diagnostic potential of CSF is great, especially in those instances where MRI spectroscopy allows for noninvasive monitoring of compounds such as *N*-acetylaspartate, choline, creatine-creatine phosphate, alanine, adenosine triphosphate (ATP), organic acids, etc. In psychiatry, the CSF has been of major interest as a gateway to transmitter metabolism in brain. Until recently, attention has centered on the monoamines and especially the association between reduced CSF 5HIAA and violence and suicide. Even beyond the questions of what kind of violence and what form of suicide are the general questions of specificity and mechanism. The concentrations of any one compound can only go up, down, or remain the same. Generally, more than one mechanism can be involved in changes in any direction. For example, a decrease can result from over-utilization as well as diminished production. Newer tools may help us arrive at the more fundamental phenomena of the mechanisms underlying the end result.

2.3.2.2.2 Animal studies. Animal studies are carried out when it is important to look at integrated biological systems rather than cellular or macromolecular responses. As in human studies, the number of subjects required is determined by the expected magnitude of the effect, the variance estimated from other studies, and the degree of acceptable statistical reliance. Again, while the number of animals should be kept to a minimum, that number should not be so small as to prevent firm conclusions if the variance is greater than expected or the mean difference between populations is smaller. Adding an extra 5 to 10% more animals to a study is reasonable. Besides the number of animals, the investigator must also decide on species, strain, sex, age, housing conditions, and treatment parameters.

Species selection is based on biological features, use in the literature, and cost. Examples of particular biological features that may be useful in specific studies include the neural reorganization between caterpillar and butterfly or tadpole and frog, mice missing a specific gene, rats developing hypertension with age, the identical offspring of the armadillo, the similarity between dog and human stomachs or pig and human hearts, or the long maturational period of marsupials. A choice must also be made between specificity and generality. There is a wealth of genetic information on many genera and especially on rodents. Some of the sites providing such genetic information are listed below. Pure strains of mice as well as knockout mice missing a specific piece of the genome are available from many sources. The results obtained with one strain, however, may not generalize to another. Rat strains are less uniform than mice strains, but rat genomics are being deciphered. Long-Evans are more difficult to handle but more alert than most others. Sprague-Dawleys are more amenable to handling. Wistars have been used in many cancer studies, as have Fischers. Beyond these differences, the same strain from different suppliers may differ. To determine the generality of a phenomenon may require replication across strains or even species. Attempts at replication require use of the same strain.

The literature also has to be considered. For example, because of the size of its brain and the hardness of its skull, the cat was an early experimental animal in neurophysiology, while size, cost, and intelligence made the rat the animal of choice for many studies on neurochemistry and physiological psychology. A study dependent on detailed anatomy may require the cat; one on neurochemistry may require the rat. Further, housing and food costs affect species selection. Large animals cost more to maintain than small ones. Depending on the question, smaller may be better for chronic longitudinal studies. Because your own studies will build upon your previous studies, the species you select at the beginning may well be with you throughout your career. Time spent selecting the appropriate species for a study is time very well spent, indeed.

The bases for deciding on sex and age are self-evident. Developmental studies require young animals, geriatric studies older ones. Male rats have the general advantage of being acyclic, but the information gained is limited to males. Studies on the female require accounting for hormonal cycles but provide information different from studies on the male.

Housing conditions also deserve some thought. Because all living creatures merit respect, laboratory animals should be as well cared for and handled as sensitively as possible within the framework of the goals of the project. This is important not only for ethical reasons but also because animals are not test tubes and their past history may affect today's behavior or biology. It is also important, therefore, to have some idea of the animal's past history. It is important to the investigator that the supplier has treated the animals humanely. Because science depends on verifiability, it is imperative that food, water, temperature, and lighting are controlled and that every effort is made to keep animals healthy and happy. It is also important to keep track of environmental variables. A drift in temperature can affect results. The timing of circadian changes in hormones, metabolic processes, activity, and body temperature is not the same on a 12:12 light:dark schedule as on a 14:10 schedule. Although standard commercial laboratory chow is pretty uniform, the alfalfa from which it is largely derived undergoes seasonal changes in plant estrogens, and water usually contains trace minerals. In most instances, these may not matter but the investigator should be aware of them. In short, animal studies, like studies on humans, require sensitivity toward the subjects and thought regarding design.

Some of the sites providing genetic information on mice, rats, and humans include:

http://ratmap.gen.gu.se/
www.informatis.jax.org
http://www.well.ok.ac.uk/
http://carbon.wi.mit.edu:8000/cgi-bin/mouse/index
http://waldo.wi.mit.edu/rat/public/

2.3.2.2.3 Neurotransmitters. There are some dozen small molecules and 50 or more peptides which are released from one neuron, bind to specific sites on another, and thus produce physiological changes. That is, they meet the criteria for neurotransmitters. Among the smaller classical transmitters the most commonly considered are serotonin, norepinephrine, epinephrine, dopamine, acetylcholine, glutamic acid, GABA, aspartic acid, glycine, histamine, adenosine, and the gas nitric oxide. Representative peptide transmitters are vasoactive intestinal polypeptide, cholecystokinin, leucine enkephalin, methionine enkephalin, substance P, neuropeptide Y, neurotensin, somatostatin, thyrotropin-releasing hormone, bombesin, luteinizing hormone-releasing hormone, adrenocorticotropic hormone, beta endorphin, vasopressin, oxytocin, galanin, and carnosine. Despite this abundance of transmitters, emphasis has been given in psychiatry to three — the monoamines serotonin, norepinephrine, and dopamine — and most current psychoactive drugs are designed to act on one or another of them.

There are two reasons for this. Working on the theory of first looking where the light is, the aromatic ring structures of the monoamines make them relatively easy to detect and quantify. Second, and perhaps more important, with few cell bodies in old regions of the brain sending long projections into the limbic structure and frontal cortex, they seem ideally suited to modulate emotional behavior, the very stuff of psychiatry. The structural similarities between various psychotomimetics and these compounds have only strengthened the general association. While the major work of the brain may be carried out by the go/no-go glutamate and gabaminergic neurons, their modulation to generate emotion is considered the work of the monoamines. Clearly, however, this is a giant simplification derived from our general ignorance. All those transmitters are not merely in the brain for stuffing but rather must also function to generate the complex images and dreams which motivate our lives. Thanks to advances in methodology, the complexity of the system is slowly coming to light.

Besides releasing a specific and characteristic classical transmitter, some neurons release a second cotransmitter, as well. Generally, but not always, this is peptide, although in some instances two classical transmitters may coexist in the same terminal. One example is the concomitant existence of the monoamines and adenosine which, in the form of its precursor ATP, is found in terminal monoamine terminal storage vesicles as an ATP-monoamine complex. There are also instances of dual peptide innervation, such as the hypothalamic neurons containing both galanin and growth hormone-releasing hormone.

These mixtures are distributed in a regionally specific manner. For example, some terminals in the mesenchephalon contain dopamine alone, while some contain both cholecystokinin and dopamine. In the hypothalamus, besides terminals with dopamine alone are some with dopamine and cholecystokinin and still others with dopamine and neurotensin. Distributions may also be transmitter specific. Neuropeptide Y does not co-localize with dopamine but does with norepinephrine in some neurons. Thyrotropic hormone is co-localized only with serotonin, but substance P is found in both some cholinergic and some serotoninergic neurons. Because many of these peptides are neurotransmitters in their own right, whether these neurons are named for the classical transmitter or the peptide is arbitrary.

The significance of co-release is complex, and a general pattern has not yet emerged. In some cases, the peptide is only released with increased firing rate and presumably serves to augment the actions of the classical transmitter. In others, the cotransmitter and transmitters seem to subserve different functions. Gender differences in cotransmitter release have also been reported, primarily for systems involved in gender-specific hormone production. And, in some cases, presynaptic stimulation increases the release of one cotransmitter while inhibiting release of the other. Most classical transmitters are synthesized locally in the neuron terminal, ready for use, but the peptide transmitters are generally produced in the cell body and shipped to the terminal. The rate of replacement for these two classes of cotransmitters, then, is quite different and so, it would be expected, would be their rate of release.

Once released, transmitters act upon receptors. If the number of transmitters is large, the number of receptors is larger still. Receptors are classified first by their natural agonist, subclassified by the metabolic consequences attendant on their binding with agonist, and further subclassified by their binding to, and interactions with, synthetic agonist and antagonists. For example, serotonergic stimulation of 5HT1 receptors inhibits adenylate cyclase, but there are currently 5HT1A, 5HT1B, 5HT1D, 5HT1E, and 5HT1F receptor sites based on interactions with synthetic ligands. On the other hand, 5HT2 sites stimulate the phosphoinositol cycle and protein kinase C and come in the two flavors of 5HT2A and 5HT2B, while 5HT3 sites open chloride channels, etc. As might be expected, the sub-subclassifications often increase with increased numbers of synthetic ligands.

The receptors themselves are complex proteins with seven transmembrane regions forming, usually, a hydrophilic binding pocket for the transmitter. While the receptors are distinct and specific for their endogenous transmitter, the structural similarities between some receptors are so marked that it would appear that one form mutated from another during the course of evolution. Most transmitters act on several receptor subtypes, and the different subtypes often have distinctive anatomical distributions.

The function of a transmitter, of course, is to convey a signal to both initiate a metabolic response and/or to continue retransmission of the signal to a more distant site. The first messenger, the transmitter, thus hands on the torch to a second messenger in the postsynaptic neuron. In the central nervous system, this is most commonly cyclic adenosine monophosphate (cAMP), or a phospholipid lipase, or direct actions on an ion channel. These metabolic messengers in turn activate protein kinase A or generate dacylglyceride, which translocates and activates protein kinase C and stimulates the phosphotidylinositol cycle to produce inositol triphosphate, which releases calcium from the endoplasmic reticulum. Increases in internal calcium, in turn, activate calcium-dependent calcium calmodulin to phosphorylate specific substrates and carry out innumerable other tasks, including some affecting transmitter synthesis, storage, and release.

The protein kinases, activated by second messengers, in turn phosphorylate serine and threonine residues on specific substrate proteins which then carry out specific cellular tasks, such as protein synthesis, translocations, transport, opening or closing channels, stimulating synthesis or assembly, etc., until dephosphorylated and inactivated by specific sets of protein phosphatases.

Psychiatric pharmacology and neurobiology have walked hand-in-hand along this line. When neurobiology focused on intermediary metabolism, pharmacology developed compounds and ways to manipulate transmitter synthesis and catabolism. When neurobiology began to examine the mechanisms for transmitter release and re-uptake, pharmacology provided the tools for these studies and developed therapies from them. Receptor binding studies led to the production of ligands stimulating or inhibiting specific transmitter-receptor interactions. Tomorrow's efforts will likely be directed at modifying the actions of second messengers and, after that, on products still further down the signaling cascade. At each step, neuropharmacology will develop many of the chemical tools needed to elucidate the neurobiology of the brain and pave the way for clinical psychiatry. Clearly, this is a very important and very active field of neurobiology and a humbling one, as well.

An excellent site for information on most of the major transmitters and peptides in brain as well as on the current status of research on psychiatric syndromes generally is

www.acnp/org/cd1998/

2.3.2.2.4 Genetics: **The human genome.** Probably the greatest modern influence on tomorrow's medicine will be medical genetics. The rapid evolution of research in this area over the past decades has fundamentally changed approaches to the pathogenesis of disease. The international Human Genome Project (HGP), designed to map and sequence the entire 3 billion base pairs on the 22 autosomes and the X and/or Y chromosomes (23 pairs), will directly link molecular genetics to disease risk with important medical consequences for therapy and identification of disease vulnerability. It may also pose important social and philosophical questions for medicine. Some of these are discussed below.

The basic plan for the genome project is deceptively simple. In essence, it consists of but three steps: (1) divide the chromosome into smaller fragments, (2) order the fragments, and (3) determine their base sequence. The Human Genome Project will also provide other data and technologies to enhance information about genes important for common complex traits in psychiatric diseases. One challenge is the further study of the functions of nonprotein-coding sequences and their effects on gene expression.

While the plan looks easy, its implementation is not. Besides the technical problems is the problem of the sheer size of the task. As indicated above, there are 3 billion base pairs to be identified. Identifying one base pair per second would take 91 years! These bases make up some 80 to 100,000 genes. Each gene, coding a single protein, is about 3000 base pairs in length; together, they code for about 80,000 different proteins. Because three bases code for one amino acid, the average of 3000 bases per gene translates into an average of 1000 amino acids per protein.

This enormous code is linear and tightly coiled in chromosomes, which are composed equally of protein and DNA. Chromosomes vary in size from the smallest, the Y chromosome, to the largest, chromosome 1. With appropriate staining, each chromosome shows a unique banding pattern, and this combination of size and banding pattern serves for chromosome identification, or karyotyping. While some of the DNA directly codes for protein (exons), most do not (introns), and although small portions of introns are involved in regulating which sections are activated, the function of most is still open.

Some current techniques use genomic DNA, consisting of both coding and "uncoding" regions. Some use cDNA, which is DNA made from the messenger RNAs formed from the protein coding regions of the genome. The technologies of gene mapping are numerous and complex. The most common are outlined here in their broadest outlines. Detailed information can be obtained at the various web sites listed below and in the many excellent texts available.

All genes are of interest to biology. Those linked to disease are of special interest to medicine. Two key concepts underlie the search for such genes. First, genomes are mixed and recombined during meosis. Second, the closer two genes are to each other the more likely they are to segregate together during recombinations. The former accounts for individuality, while the ease of segregation has been used to estimate genetic distance in terms of Morgans (M). That is, one centimorgan (about 1 million base pairs in physical distance) is defined as the distance separating two genes that have a 1% recombination rate.

The task, then, is to identify a genetic abnormality which tracks with the disease, isolate it, and determine its sequence and mode of action so that it can be either ultimately replaced with an intact gene or, more often, normal function restored by some therapeutic maneuver. The recombinations of genomes and mutations are such that a single nucleotide difference between individuals occurs in about every 100 to 300 base pairs. Most of these are on introns. These single nucleotide polymorphisms (SNP) and variable numbers of short repeated nucleotide sequences (tandem repeats) are used as markers in gene mapping and also serve in the hunt for genetic abnormalities.

The first step is to localize the region with the defective gene. This requires identifying families with a high incidence of inherited disease and obtaining tissue from afflicted and normal members of the family. The tissue is usually either skin or blood. The former is used for fibroblasts, the latter to obtain nucleated lymphocytes which can then be immortalized by infecting them with the Epstein-Barr virus (EBV). The cells are then cultured to obtain sufficient DNA for extraction, purification, and analysis. Usually the entire cellular DNA is extracted, but (more recently) the DNA from specific chromosomes can also be identified by size and laser-analyzed DNA and sorted by flow cytometry. The DNA is then cut using bacterial-derived restriction enzymes (RE) as scissors. There are many available restriction enzymes, each of which selectively cuts the DNA at specific nucleotide sequences.

The size of the resultant DNA pieces increases sharply with the number of nucleotides required by the recognition site of the enzyme. Enzymes requiring four base sites, for example, yield fragments of about 250 bases, while those only recognizing specific strings of eight bases produce fragments 64,000 bases long. In general, segments of 100 to 500 base pairs are often used to examine for genetic disease. The cut pieces are then sorted and sized, usually by gel electrophoresis. Because of the minuscule amounts of material involved, sensitive fluorescent or radioactive techniques may be used to identify them, and the fragments appear as lines, much like those on a bar code. Any differences between individuals in the specific nucleotide sequence in the recognition site of the particular restriction enzyme used will prevent cleavage. This will result in a difference in the size of the resultant fragments. Abnormal bands can then be excised and amplified either by cloning (incorporating the band into the genetic structure of a vector such as bacteriophage which in turn infects a bacteria and forces it to produce large amounts of the protein of interest) or by using the polymerase chain reaction (PCR), if part of its nucleotide sequence is known. The goal in both cases is to obtain enough material to sequence.

The nucleotide fragment obtained by all this is unlikely to be the aberrant gene itself but rather something sufficiently close to it to segregate with it and be useful as a marker. It can be used to identify the approximate chromosomal region carrying the abnormality, the degree of its segregation among family members providing a clue as to its proximity to the disease gene. Location can be further narrowed with other markers on the chromosome. Once localized between two known markers, the intervening area can be sequenced and the diseased gene identified. Then comes the search for its function and for ways to circumvent its pathological effect.

As one can see, this is a complex task. Genes are small and regions large. Single-base defects causing disease (probably the case for most human inherited diseases) are currently not possible to find by this process alone. It helps if some information already exists on pharmacological responses or on associated biochemical abnormalities, for these implicate candidate genes to examine first. An example, again, is phenylketonuria. The increase in blood phenylalanine in this disease led to finding the defective gene product in liver phenylalanine hydroxylase. Identification of the normal enzyme and its amino acid sequence would materially help in locating possible genetic sites and, thereby, in locating the defective gene. Indeed, in general, mapping the entire gene is easier than finding a specific single base genetic defect.

While genomic mapping also involves splitting, ordering, and sequencing DNA fragments, its goal is to detail the haystack rather than the needles lost within it. And the many techniques that have evolved to facilitate genomic mapping, while applicable to the search for genetic disease, do not always touch the central problem. Thus, besides using polymorphisms and repeats as markers, the order and distance between markers can be adduced by the linkages remaining after chromosomal fragmentation following *in vitro* radiation. Larger and larger fragments of DNA, some as large as 1 Mb, can be cloned as artificial chromosomes in yeast. Pulse-field electrophoretic methods permit separation of very large DNA fragments. Improvements in fluorescent techniques and *in situ* hybridization procedures enormously increase the resolution for mapping of genomic sites. Also, direct identification of nucleotides by spectrophotometric, fluorescent, and scanning tunneling microscopy has speeded the time required for sequencing the enormous number of bases in the human gene. While these techniques may not help much with a single gene search, once the genomic maps are complete, finding and decoding mutations of those hidden needles will be easier by making markers of all genes. It is important to find them not only to provide reliable genetic, metabolic, immunologic, or neurologic criteria for an etiological diagnosis but also because they may predict pharmacogenetic and pharmacogenomic research strategies for more effective treatment.

There are two parts to pharmacogenetic analyses: pharmacokinetics and pharmacodynamics. Pharmacokinetics deals with the absorption, distribution, first liver passage, and general metabolism and elimination of drugs. Transport processes in the epithelia of different organs and drug-metabolizing enzymes such as the cytochrome P450 system are under genetic control. Genetic variations in these systems profoundly affect the pharmacokinetics of many psychoactive drugs.

Pharmacodynamics deals with the relationship between the concentration of a drug and the response at its site of action which, for neuropsychiatry, includes neurotransmitter receptors and transporters. Genetic variation also plays a role in the drug-induced neuronal plasticity that occurs on long-term treatment with psychoactive drugs. Increased information and understanding of pharmacogenetics will benefit rational drug design, the detection of genetic predispositions to disease, tendencies to addiction, and the risks for side effects from medications, such as the dyskinesia following some antipsychotic drugs. While many genetic diseases result from single gene mutations, some may instead be due to the nexus of susceptibilities. Such polygenic diseases pose additional problems for genetic identification and require more information on the interaction between genetic propensities and environmental exposures over the entire life span.

Indeed, most, perhaps all, psychiatric disorders do involve a complex interplay between genetic and environmental factors. The importance of environmental stimuli in initiating and/or exacerbating psychiatric disease has been well documented. Clearly, etiological research into these complex disorders and the environments affecting symptom expression raises many sociological and political, as well as clinical, questions. Elucidating that interaction will require not only genetic information but also information on the neurochemical and neurophysiological effects of perceived environmental change. In addition, the deciphering will require application of such statistical tools as survival analysis to estimate morbid risk, structural equation models for partitioning phenotypic variances and covariances into component genetic and environmental influences, complex segregation analysis to detect loci of major effect, and linkage and association analysis for the localization and identification of susceptibility genes.

Among the many web sites dealing with the Human Genome Project and genomics in general are

> **www.ncbi.nlm.nih.gov/genome/guide/**
> **www.ncbi.nlm.nih.gov/disease/Brain.html**
> **www.ncbi.nlm.nih.gov/Omim/Stats/mimstats.html**
> **www.ornl.gov/hgmis/pblicat/primer/prim2.htm**
> **www.bioscience.igh.cnrs.fr//urllists/genemap.htm**

www.pedgen.med.uni-muenchen.de/medgen/databases.html
www.uwcm.ac.uk/uwcm/mg/psychemap/
www.nlm.nih.gov/genemap/
www.ncbi.nlm.nih.gov/Web/Genbank/index.html
www-bli.unizh.ch/BLI/Projects/genetics/K225.html
www.genome.wi.mit.edu
www.nimh.nih.gov/studies/index.cfm
www.ornl.gov/TechResources/Human_Genome/publicat/
   publications.html
www.ddbj.nig.ac.jp/
www.genome.ad.jp/kegg/kegg.html
www.agrf.org.au
www.angris.org.au

Ethical issues. The ultimate success of the Human Genome Project will raise a number of social and psychiatric issues. We have just emerged from a period of simplistic belief that environment is everything, only to enter one of simplistic belief that the gene is everything. The reality that both are important, that they interact, and that we as individuals have minimal control over either should not be ignored.

The shining promise of genetic medicine has already brought great benefits to medicine but it also poses some obvious dangers. Elucidating human genomic structure will permit medicine, at long last, to prevent and circumvent genetic diseases. Without gene ablation and replacement, however, the successful treatment of genetic diseases also permits dissemination of those genes into wider and wider populations. It is therefore important that the general public, and especially potential parents, be given full access to professional genetic counseling.

Similarly, increased knowledge regarding the control of cell death and cell replacement has the potential of immeasurably extending human life, but, with that extension, it also carries the risk of further increasing all the dangers of overpopulation. In nations where access to medical treatment is controlled by insurers, genetic information may be misused to inversely relate access and risk rather than directly relate them as in classical medicine. The ability to modify genetic makeup may lead to pressure on physicians by potential parents to select for offspring with special phenotypes or may be misused by nations to breed "ideal" soldiers. That pressure has already led to the marketing of "choice" eggs and sperm, and theories of genetic differences have led to much human misery.

It is a biological truism that, while survival of the individual is best when it approximates the population mean, survival of the species requires the widest possible gene pool. What will be needed for survival today may not be what is required tomorrow.

It is hoped that the study of genetics will provoke debates on free will and determinism, on genetic selection, on potential immortality, and on the science-fiction ideas of designing bodies to survive on other planets, as well as leading to an acceptance of our fellow human beings. Individuals cannot select their own parents, their own gene structures, or even the environment in which they were born, yet all affect an individual's life. With knowledge comes power, and with more knowledge comes increased tolerance.

chapter three

Results

3.1 General comments

This is not a textbook on statistics nor can it substitute for the insights of a real live statistician. Your study probably requires input from a statistician if: (1) you are dealing with complex, marginal, or infrequent events; (2) you are studying populations where relevant variables cannot be controlled; (3) you are trying to examine for interactions between variables; (4) you are looking at many variables at a time; (5) you are looking for small changes in the midst of much noise; or (6) you are looking for a needle in a haystack.

There are, of course, numerous other situations when you should consider consulting a statistician, as well. Nearly all studies on human populations require some statistical help because of the many relevant variables that cannot be controlled and because the sample studied may differ from the general population. If there are multiple variables, the chance of finding a difference by chance increases and requires different statistical procedures than those necessary to handle a single variable. You might also need a statistician if some of your data are parametric and some are not and you are not sure how to combine them. You need a statistician if your data set has missing data and when you decide, with the statistician, whether to fill the missing slots by carrying the last value forward, by using the mean of the two adjacent values, or by substituting the mean for all values. Repeated measures in longitudinal studies must be treated differently than single variables in a parallel comparison. Indeed, it is a good idea to consult a statistician even if you do not think you need one, and it is good to do so before the study begins rather than afterwards. Most statisticians are pretty insightful about number problems and are adept at detecting and identifying problems that will bedevil you later. They often also have very good suggestions on how to get the maximum information from the minimum sample size. And do not be surprised if two expert statisticians disagree. Statisticians, like clinicians or any other experts, have their own views about the best way to approach a problem, and while they agree on simple problems they may differ on more complex ones.

3.2   *Data handling*

Data can accumulate at a very rapid rate, especially if you are industrious and/or are looking at many variables; therefore, it is imperative that you devise some routine for tabulating and filing incoming data before they swamp you. Because data come in all shapes, sizes, and forms, no single method may work for all situations. There are some general considerations, however. Experiments have to be identified; so do tests, and so do subjects. Besides a title, the experiment should be given a unique number, letter, or alphanumeric identification. Numbers have the advantage of going on forever. They have the disadvantage that subject number and experiment number might get confused. Three letters are limited to only 17,576 combinations (13,824 if Q and U are eliminated) but cannot be confused with subject number. Alphanumeric combinations combine the advantages of both systems. Whatever the decision, a hardbacked or loose-leaf notebook should be set aside as a central hard-copy experiment index that lists the identification and title of each experiment. It is worth having even if another copy is kept on the hard drive of your computer or on a separate floppy disk. This index could also contain information on the location of subsets of the data or even summaries of the data, although such summaries may become impossibly bulky. The advantage of the index is that it provides easy access for study and assessment of progress. You can take it to the bathroom, which you cannot do with the computer. Often it is better to keep summaries of the data, the actual data, and/or information on the location of relevant data in separate notebooks and/or computer files identified by experiment title and identification number. All data related to the experiment should also be marked with the experiment identification number, its own identification, and subject identification. For example, a Hamilton rating scale for subject 12 in experiment ABC might be identified as ABC12Hamilton or ABC12H. This system allows for some sorting if there is misfiling or other displacement of the data.

A filing system can also help when the time comes to write up the study. The process can be simplified if the experimental design, experimental methods, and summaries of the data are kept together in a notebook and/or computer file along with relevant literature articles. Indeed, it often helps focus a study if the introduction and methods sections of one or more papers expected to result from the data are written early in the study, well before the data are collected. Not only can this focus the study, but the very fact that the documents exist makes writing the rest of the paper easier. And, of course, the documents can be modified as necessary, if the data drive the work in a different direction.

The experiment will create a plethora of data, and the raw data from which all else is derived should be kept in hard copy in the experiment notebook. The workup of the data, however, will generally also create a plethora of computer files. A running notebook of file genealogy and definitions of acronyms may help prevent madness, especially when, months later, a reviewer raises a question and you cannot remember the location of the files or the acronym assigned to the data. Suppose, for example, that a portion of a data file on the total population called ABCT was used to create another file on depressives in the sample which was then labeled ABCD. Now suppose that this data file, in turn, was used as the input for an analysis of variance which was identified as ACBDV. A genealogy of the sequence might look like this: ABCT > ABCD > ACBDV.

3.3 *Data analysis*

The first thing to do with raw data is to look at the data before further processing. In addition to looking at the data at the end of the study — if the study is not double blind, or if you are not involved in both gathering and analyzing the data, or if the data are generated by procedures that you cannot in any way influence — also examine the data over the entire course of the experiment. How variable are the numbers? Do the numbers or does variance change over time? Are there crazy numbers that could be transcription errors? Are one or two values widely different from the others? If you have enough data, plot a histogram; that is, divide the values into equal ranges and plot the number of data points in each range against the mean value of the range. Is the distribution bell-shaped with a single peak and nearly equal populations on both sides of the peak, or is it skewed with the bulk of the population of numbers on one side of the peak? If you have the means and standard errors of many measures, do the standard errors increase with increasing means? Are there missing data? How much? If it is a drug study and people have dropped out, did they drop out because they died or because the side effects outweighed the gain or because they all got well? If it is necessary to fill in the missing values, will you carry the last value forward, substitute the mean for that individual, or take the average of the two adjacent values?

The reason for going through all this is so that you will be warned of problems before going to the trouble of data analysis and before data analysis obscures the problem. It is discouraging after a long analysis to discover that the gigantic difference in the means of two populations is only due to the error of transcribing the decimal place on some samples or to learn that the terrific correlation you hoped for is due only to two extreme numbers which do not represent the sample. A close look at the data could also indicate the need to recheck or re-analyze data. If the numbers are very variable, is it because of variance in the assay or within subjects or between subjects? When it is possible to do so, re-evaluating some subjects with the highest and lowest values or re-analyzing the samples can be both comforting and informative. If the data shift with time or if the first collected data look different than the last collected data for subjects who should be comparable, then the measurements might not be stable or the subjects might not be stable. For example, raters using a rating form may unknowingly change their criteria over time, or the sensitivity of an instrument may change as its photomultiplier tube ages, or the first data may have been collected from eager volunteers and the last from subjects recruited for a fee, etc. Whatever the situation, a shift in the numbers over time is a warning that should not be ignored.

Unique data points separated from other data points are called "outliers." Depending on circumstances, such numbers can introduce variance sufficient to hide real differences between populations or may indicate a difference where one really does not exist. The great problem is in deciding if an outlier is representative of the sample examined, if it is from another population, or if it is due to some error. In the first case, the outlier must be included in the sample. In the second case, the outlier should be discarded or made part of a different sample. Finally, if the outlier is due to an error, it must surely be discarded. The usual test of whether an outlier is within the tested population is to recalculate the mean and standard deviation for the sample without the variant number. If the variant number is now more than 2 standard deviations from the recalculated mean, the variant number should be discarded from the sample. This test is based on the fact that 2 standard deviations encompass 99% of all values in a Gaussian distribution. Anything outside that range is regarded as coming from another population of numbers and is discarded. An alternate procedure is to apply the Trimmed or Wilcoxen T-test whereby highest and lowest values in each population are replaced by their next highest and lowest numbers. Alternate versions trim the population of numbers by a set percentage. Wilcoxen T-tables substitute for Student T-tables in assessing significance using these procedures. All methods are based on the premise of obtaining a mean value more representative of the population examined.

A shift in numbers can also occur by chance. As every gambler knows, Lady Luck sometimes smiles and sometimes frowns. Correspondingly, by chance, there will be bunches of highly sensitive or insensitive subjects or animals who will produce data quantitatively different than that of the total sample. Because any chance event is unrelated to preceding or past events, such strings may not be matched by equal strings in the opposite direction. That is, a flip of 10 heads in a row is unlikely to be followed (ever) by a flip of 10 tails in a row. As a result, adding more samples may dilute, but may not otherwise normalize, the data. It is for this reason, among many others, that it is important to replicate studies.

Transcription errors are always a problem. Whenever possible two people should recheck numbers rather than one, just as two people should proof a paper rather than one. It is amazing how easy it is for the eye of one observer to misread the same thing twice. If the data are not Gaussian in distribution or if the magnitude of the standard errors correlates with the magnitude of the mean, the usual statistical treatments may give misleading results. Either non-Gaussian statistical procedures should be used, or the data should be transformed into a form more Gaussian in distribution before analysis. Taking the log of the value or the square root of the number will often produce a more Gaussian distribution. It should be noted that biological data are often non-Gaussian in distribution, and calculating the raw numbers may provide different results than using the normalized values.

Much more trivial is the question of whether the number of digits in the data is meaningful. For example, suppose that the mean of a set of rating scale numbers is to be used as a data point and the numbers are 1, 3, 5, 7, 2, 6, 9. The mean is 3.2857142... . However, the component numbers themselves are no better than 1 part in 10, and the mean should not be entered as more precise than 3.3, or one part in 33. Not only do the larger numbers of digits increase transcribing errors, but they also simply add noise to the results.

Finally, turn the same critical eye on the transformed data. Computational errors occur in computer programs as well as in hand calculations. Keyboard errors can occur as do program errors. This is evident even today in the many news stories on computer errors in banking, billing, and space probes.

3.4 Statistical treatments

Don't be overwhelmed by statistical manipulations. Statistics were born to help gamblers assess the odds of winning or losing.

Statistics are used in science to assess the odds of being right or wrong. They are not a guarantee of either. Statistics simply allow investigators to hedge their bets. The 0.05 level of significance merely means that you have one chance in 20 of being wrong. It does not mean you are right. And, indeed, at some time, you are likely to be wrong, 0.05 or not. Ten separate, careful experiments testing a hypothesis with different techniques and arriving at the same conclusions are more convincing than a single experiment, no matter the statistical significance. It should also be clear that statistical significance may not translate into clinical significance. A statistically significant change may occur in one variable in a set which has no relevance to the course of the disease, treatment response, or recovery. Indeed, the literature is full of comparisons, often carried out between competing drug houses, each attempting to show how its drug is better than other drugs on one or another variable. Often these variables are of minor clinical significance. Further, remember that an experiment with many comparisons is likely to find differences due to chance alone. Paired comparisons on 100 variables will, on average, yield by chance one difference at $p < 0.01$ and five at $p < 0.05$. A number of multiple-range tests — the Duncan or the Bonferonni, for example — account for multiple variable tests, but, even so, chance differences slip by. Indeed, multivariate experiments can often be regarded as pilot experiments that identify variables that should be further tested for validity.

Three factors are critical to any comparison: the size of the signal, the noise level, and the number of observations. It is difficult to recognize a low tone in the midst of loud, roaring traffic. It is easy to do so in a quiet room. A fourth factor, the desired degree of certainty in the conclusions, must be added for statistical comparisons. If the signal is large and the variance small enough, the number of replications necessary to assert a difference is small. The difference in height between a human and an ant is so large and the relative variance so small that a single set of measurements would suffice to assert that humans are taller than ants and very few more measurements to assert that finding with a $p < 0.001$. Similarly, if drug X cured all treated subjects but drug Y left them all sick, only a small number of subjects would be required to conclude that drug X is better than drug Y. In most of psychiatry, however, effects of therapies are seldom so dramatic or variance so low, so correspondingly larger numbers of subjects are required to test for statistical differences in relative efficacy. Often one can do little to change the magnitude of the effect. Frequently, though, a great deal can be done to decrease variance and thereby the number of subjects necessary for study. That is, such things as ambiguities in rating scales, variations between raters, shifts in ratings over time, insensitive or unspecific measures, uneven distributions of characteristics in the populations studied, and external interference during testing periods all add to statistical noise. Many of these can be minimized to decrease the number of subjects necessary for the study. There are, of course, trade-offs. For example, decreasing population heterogeneity by limiting it to one gender, one age group, one level of severity, or some other measure may decrease the sample size at the expense of decreasing the generality of results. Conversely, increased inclusion increases the number of needed subjects. Generally, however, the effort spent increasing the magnitude of the signal or, more often, decreasing the statistical noise is more than repaid in the clarity of the results. In any event, determining the population size required to test for an effect at some level of statistical significance is of considerable importance. Too often studies are carried out and reported such that a reader cannot tell if a negative result means "no" or "undetermined." Such ambiguity confuses, not clarifies, and should be assiduously avoided. In science, it is better to know what you do not know than to be uncertain.

Finally, it must be stressed that correlations and statistical relationships alone do not necessarily demonstrate causation. Nor should a statistical relationship be taken out of context or overinterpreted. Thus, the statistical fact that more people in America die in the hospital than die at home is more likely to mean that very sick people go to hospitals than that American hospitals are life threatening. Similarly, a positive correlation between the size of child's head and performance on a spelling test may merely reflect age-dependent changes in both. A statistically significant correlation between the number of telephones and the number of births should not be interpreted to mean telephones produce babies but rather may mean no more than that telephones facilitate arranging meetings between boys and girls.

Unexpected relationships, though, should not necessarily be passed off as coincidence. Events seemingly improbable upon calculation are not improbable at all. For example, there is a better than even chance that two people in a group of 23 will have the same birth date, and a 70% probability if the group number exceeds 30. Gamblers and magicians thrive on the probability of the seemingly improbable, and a little calculation can go a long way. In all events, however, statistics are a tool to be used by the head and not as a substitute for it.

There is an enormous number of statistical resources on the web. Just using the term "statistics" with any search engine will turn up a plethora of sites. Three particularly useful sites with lots of links are

http://www.stat.ufl.edu/vlib.statistics.html
http://www.statsol.com/tools/stattools/
http://members.aol.com/johnp71/javastat.htm

chapter four

Appendix

4.1 How to read a paper

Indicus Medicus currently abstracts some 3200 journals of medical interest. Medline covers 4300, and these are only the more important journals. *Science Citation Index*, covering all of science, lists 8500 journals. It is no wonder that the average physician feels overwhelmed, and it will only get worse. Free journals fill mailboxes. Pharmaceutical houses provide reprints favorable to their products along with lunches, seminars, pens, and other little gifts. Every major organization publishes a journal, often including the cost of it in membership dues. Other prestigious journals overflow library shelves. Only the cost of journals has limited the number of available journals in most libraries but, as more journals go onto the Internet, this limit, too, will vanish. What, then, should a poor physician do?

Why read the literature at all, though? The answer is simple. Medicine changes daily, and not reading the literature puts patients at risk. A physician today with yesterday's ideas is a menace. Yet, journals must be read with care and understanding if the information is to do any good.

The first decision to be made is deciding what is important to know at the moment. The second is deciding where to find it. And, once found, it is essential to understand what the information really means.

Journals are read mostly to keep up with new treatments, prognostic indicators, and information on the etiology of disorders. Sometimes the literature is necessary to develop the background for a new study or sometimes for the details of a required methodology. Occasionally, it is even perused out of simple curiosity, or as bathroom reading, or just to while away the hours. In all these cases, it is usually the title, the authors' names, the research site, and the abstract which determine whether the rest of the paper gets read. As noted in the next section, it is therefore critical that authors pay attention to all three of these components in their own manuscript.

Once a purpose for reading has been established, the next question becomes where to look among these thousands of sources. Not all journals are equal. The editor, the editorial board, and the quality of reviewers' comments have made some journals more prestigious than others. The better journals often stay better because they get more submissions and can thereby be more selective. Rankings do change along with editors and editorial boards, and any listing here might be misleading tomorrow; however, there is a rough correlation between a journal's standing and the number of times it is cited in the literature. Yearly tabulations are found in various places, such as the *Science Citation Index*. Electronic publication, at least at the beginning, will still maintain this editorial structure. With time, however, it may very well vanish, making it all the more imperative that the reader can efficiently discard inadequate studies.

Currently, articles come in two flavors: peer reviewed and accepted without review. While important articles may appear in non-peer-reviewed journals, don't bet on it. Most are printed to support the views of the editor, publisher, or a major advertiser and are often no more than technical advertisements. The average physician's mail is flooded with them.

How long the distinction between peer-reviewed and non-peer-reviewed articles prevails, however, is uncertain, given the rapid movement toward electronic publication. Some suggest that peer-reviewed and non-peer-reviewed contributions should continue to be so identified in electronic presentations, while others argue they should not. The argument that they should be identified rests on the importance of peer review in assuring some degree of competence in the investigation and validity of the findings. To abandon peer review, proponents argue, is to abandon the utility of the literature. Those on the other side point to the time required for peer review and note that many papers do not pass this screening that may yet be important. Whatever happens in the future, over the short term, at least, electronic publishing will be tied to journals and undergo a journal peer-review process.

All peer-reviewed articles go through a similar screening process. Only the quality and the available space for publication differ. This space will greatly expand on the Internet. Some chief editors of peer-reviewed journals, along with one or more associate editors, read the manuscripts before sending them out to two or more independent reviews. Some editors send them out to be reviewed directly. The chief editor then evaluates the reviewers' comments and based on them either decides on publication or, if the reviews are in fundamental conflict, sends the article out to other reviewers for further review.

In all cases, the reviewer's job is to evaluate the importance of the manuscript and to ensure that it is appropriate to the journal, that it meets the standard for scientific competence, and that the presentation is clear. More often than not, the reviewer's recommendations require some changes in even acceptable manuscripts, which are then returned to the authors for revision before resubmission and re-evaluation. All this takes time, but if the reviewers really do their job, the reader ends up with reasonably important papers in which the subjects and the methods are clearly defined and the conclusions are commensurate with that data. Without such screening, none of these attributes is likely to be present. And, of course, the more heavily screened an article is, the more time the process takes. A good paper in a very respected journal generally takes at least a third longer to get published than a paper in a second-rate journal. Electronic publication will not speed this process. The rate-limiting steps are the time for review and the time for revision. Expert reviewers are unpaid and invariably busy, which is why they are expert in the first place. Reviewing the papers of others is seldom on top of their priority list despite the best editorial exhortations. Electronic publishing, however, can materially decrease the four months or so required to get an accepted manuscript into print.

Literature reviews are in a more ambiguous category than articles. Some are peer reviewed but most are solicited. Reputable journals such as *Schizophrenia Research, FASEB Journal,* and the *Journal of Biological Chemistry* invite reviews on specific topics from experts in the field to help keep their readers current. Such reviews, of course, beyond some human bias, are reasonably objective and informative. They are invaluable when first entering a field. Some corporations also solicit expert reviews in selected areas of corporate interest. Many of these are also very useful. Some, however, try to appear objective but are slanted toward a particular view or product. Generally, these are easily recognized and should be read with caution.

Finally, there are Letters to the Editor. Besides their gossip value, such letters sometimes usefully warn of possible side effects, identify unique problems, and raise issues and questions about preceding articles or about the field in general. Some are sufficiently important to prompt larger, more definitive studies. Such observations are growing in number and importance with electronic information flow.

It is an old scientific adage that, "Conclusions giveth but the methods taketh away." Accordingly, the methods section of an article should be the first examined after the title and abstract have stimulated serious interest. It may save much time, for if the population, the method of study, the adequacy of the tests employed, and the methods of analysis are unsatisfactory, the reader need not bother reading the remainder of the article.

Among the questions to ask about a study on diagnosis or a diagnostic test is whether the experimental populations fairly represent those proposed to suffer from the same disease. That is, diagnosis should be linked to etiology even if etiology is unknown. Is evaluation carried out blind to diagnosis? Is the control population, if one is used, demographically similar to the experimental population? Are the two populations matched for such factors as physical impairment or incarceration or are factors such as these controlled in some other manner? What criteria are used to assess the validity of the proposed diagnostic tool? Is the proposed procedure easier to apply and more predictive of disease onset, severity, incidence, course, or therapeutic response than existing procedures? Does it have predictable consequences? Is the method of analysis appropriate for the methodology? As discussed previously, congruence with a communication diagnosis may be inadequate to establish an alternative diagnostic test.

The situation is somewhat different when evaluating the results of a therapy. The usual design for such studies is to compare the efficacy of the treatment either against another treatment or against placebo. First, look for the nature of the sample. A study on the elderly may not be relevant to one interested in pediatrics. Next, look to see if subjects were randomly assigned to treatment groups or, if not, whether they were first paired on medically relevant measures to assure equal numbers in each group and then randomly assigned. If neither, proceed with caution. Third, were all clinically relevant outcomes reported and were all patients entering the study accounted for? Attrition, the bane of the statistician, is almost inevitable in any large study requiring informed consent, and all studies must have informed consent. Subjects drop out for a variety of reasons. It is important to identify those reasons that are clinically relevant, and it is especially important to know if attrition was due to side effects, death, or recovery. If a large fraction of the entering population drops out from the study and the reasons are not given, little information about therapeutic benefit can be drawn from the remainder. Next, look for how the missing data were handled. Was the analysis limited only to those who completed the study, without comment on those who did not? Was the analysis limited to the period before dropouts? Was that time sufficient for a therapeutic response? If the study extended for some time and there were dropouts, were the values assigned the dropouts the last measure carried forward, or was the mean value for the set used, or the mean of two adjacent values? Each of these issues weights the final result in a somewhat different way.

Assuming that the sample is of interest, that groups were randomly assigned, that missing data were adequately treated, and that the reasons for dropouts are given, look next at the number of subjects. In accordance with the previous discussion on the linkage between the size of the effect, the variance, and the number of subjects, a very large subject population often indicates the authors expected only a marginal therapeutic effect. In this, therapeutic studies differ from epidemiological ones, for in the latter large populations are sought primarily to obtain generality. In the therapeutic trial, a large population is often used merely to gain statistical significance. Also, look for the number of variables analyzed. If that number is also large, beware. What the conclusions giveth may be no more than an effect that is marginal in magnitude and possibly due to chance alone. And, in all events, ask yourself if the results are clinically as well as statistically significant. The two need not be equivalent, and in many studies they are not. Indeed, many equally effective drugs do differ in relatively minor, but statistically significant ways. Finally, see if the follow-up period was sufficient to detect long-term untoward effects. If all subjects improve after two weeks of treatment but drop dead after eight, a two-week rating is more than misleading. Only if the methods seem adequate should you continue on to results and discussion.

Prognosis and information on disease course are inexorably linked, but good information regarding disease course is often very difficult to come by, for what is needed is an inception cohort. A hospital population consists of those ill enough to require hospitalization and able enough to get it. The often-cited example is that of victims of heart attack. Those who reach the hospital represent the 50% who survive. These patients likely differ from those who did not. Information on the course of their disease drawn from this sample of survivors, then, may not be applicable to the entire sample and may thereby be misleading. In the case of psychiatric illnesses, it is difficult to know whether an increased incidence in something is due to increased medical availability and medical reporting or an actual increase in incidence. Schizophrenic symptoms may be well tolerated in one environment but not another, and estimates of disease incidence and course may be correspondingly colored. And, obviously, if the course of the disease is to be defined, complete follow-up is essential. The most critical questions, then, are how was the sample collected and for how long was the study carried out? Retrospective studies especially require careful scrutiny, as they are usually carried out on a hospitalized subpopulation, which may be particularly vulnerable to disease. For example, estimating the severity and probability of reoccurrence of depression in the general population from a study on hospitalized depressives risks overestimating severity and underestimating single occurrences.

In summary, the critical things to look at in the methods section before proceeding with the rest of the article are the methods for subject recruitment and subject assignment, the validity and reliability of the measures or the procedures used to assure them, and the adequacy of the analysis, number of subjects, and number of variables. If these are not satisfactory, you may be wasting your time reading further, as you will not be able to draw reliable conclusions from the data in the tables and figures.

A list of on-line journals can be found at:

http://highwire.stanford.edu

4.2   How to write a paper

You have completed your study, analyzed your data, and now know something no one else in the whole world knows. Because that something may be of use to others, you want to communicate it. Now you must answer the following questions.

4.2.1   Where

Journals differ in what they publish and the format required. Information about both appears as "Instructions to Authors," usually on the first or last page of each volume or in the first or last volume of the year. The same information can also be obtained by writing to the editorial office of the journal. Include a self-addressed, stamped envelope when you inquire. It is often useful to make, and periodically update, a folder of these instructions for the journals that you plan to use.

Journal formats primarily differ only with regard to how references are handled. Some journals prefer to cite authors in the text by number, others by author and date. Correspondingly, the bibliography may list references alphabetically or in order of appearance. Because you will cite the work of many authors, keep the entire reference of each citation (authors, title, journal, volume, inclusive page numbers, and year) in the appropriate place in the text until you decide which journal you plan to use. This is especially useful if you are writing a review or if you are submitting to a journal that identifies references by number in the text and bibliography rather than by author and date. It is easy to mix up the numbers if you insert or delete a reference or two as you write. It is also useful to keep a full copy of the paper, including the extended references, on file until after it is reviewed by the journal. A reviewer may suggest changes requiring additional references, thereby altering the number sequence. Having the full format is also useful if you submit to another journal that uses a different format. Some computer reference programs will do this for you; however, because the references get in the way of reading and editing the text, you may want to keep both a fully referenced and reduced reference version of the paper on file.

Journals do differ in prestige, largely reflecting the quality and policies of their editors and reviewers. Because prestigious journals receive the greatest number of papers, they are the most selective and have the highest rejection rates. Rankings change with time, new editors, and new reviewers. You may as well try for the best, but if your paper is rejected, the reviewer's comments may help you make the study or the presentation better. Look over recent issues of journals in your area to see which is most likely to accept your kind of study.

4.2.2   Who

The list of authors identifies those responsible for the content and ideas of the work. Authorship on papers is also important to personal advancement. To minimize conflicts, it is useful to carry out early discussions with all those involved in the study regarding duties, authorship, and order of authors. Authors are generally ordered on a paper according to their contributions to the study. The first or senior author is generally the one with prime responsibility for the work and usually is the one who conceived of the study and did most of the work, including writing the paper. If the paper issues from a major laboratory, the last author is often the head of that laboratory and the one who assumes major responsibility for the validity of the paper.

It is easier to say who should be an author than who should not. An author should make a substantial contribution to the paper beyond carrying out a routine activity. Among the authors should be anyone who raised the idea of the study, devised specific procedures outside the existing literature which were necessary to carry out the study, interpreted the data, or integrated the data into the existing literature. Acknowledgment should be given to those who make such substantive but routine contributions to the project as carrying out established assays, typing or proofing the paper, or reading the paper and making general suggestions for its improvement. Often the lines are not clear, and the senior author — usually the one who conceived of the project in the first place — makes the decisions. However, the senior author should be open to the views of anyone who can present evidence of substantive, non-routine contributions. When collaborators make equal contributions, the order of authors can be alphabetical, established by some random process such as a throw of the dice, or by rotating the order on a series of papers. In such cases, it is appropriate to indicate the procedure in a footnote. In all events, it is good to include a footnote listing the authors and their separate contributions to the paper.

4.2.3   When

A scientific project, like any work of art, is never completed but is merely abandoned. There is always more to do, and the point of abandonment is arbitrary. An appropriate stopping point is when at least one clear answer or one clear fact has been obtained. Papers are most clear if they address one question at a time. If your data provide answers to multiple questions, multiple papers are justified. Do not, however, write multiple half-papers if one will do, even though they may fill your *curriculum vitae* faster. It is not good for science, and, ultimately, it will not be good for you.

4.2.4   How

Actually, you know how to write a paper. You have by now read a host of them in the process of formulating your study, again in finding methods, and yet again in trying to put the material together. You know that the general format for almost all journals consists of: introduction, methods and materials, results, and discussion. Further, you know by example what goes into each of these categories. Everything below, then, is simply a recapitulation of what you know, with perhaps a helpful hint or two thrown in.

4.2.4.1   Introduction

Introductions are difficult only because they are at the beginning and beginnings are difficult. Actually, though, it is the easiest part of a paper, because you know why you did the study and you know the background material from which it arose. You may have to do a more recent literature search to make sure you are up to date, but, beyond that, you need merely move from the general to the specific, from the status of the field to your specific problem and approach. Among the infinite ways to do this is to start with some phrase such as, "Recent studies have shown that..." followed by "However,..." or "This implies that..." followed by "We therefore undertook... ."

4.2.4.2   Methods and materials

This, too, is an easy section. You know what you did, and here you merely report it. However, science relies on replication, and the reporting should be sufficiently detailed so as to permit replication. Try not to frustrate the reader the same way as you were frustrated when the paper you were reading left out the most critical information needed. In a clinical study, make sure the subjects, including controls, are defined both clinically and demographically so well that analogous populations could be gathered by others. Mention any environmental factors (temperature, lighting, season, diet) that could affect the results. If complex routines are involved, you may want to provide an outline. Do not refer to unpublished methods or procedures. They are of no value to the reader and your purpose should be to inform, not impress. At the least, provide enough detail of the unpublished method to permit replication even if you have a more detailed accounting in press somewhere else. List the source of any materials that are not routinely available or when differences in the products of different suppliers might influence the results. Also, indicate how the data were handled and refer to any statistical procedures you may have used. In general, if you write with the kind of detail you would like to see in a study that you might wish to replicate, you cannot go wrong.

4.2.4.3   Results

Once more, this should be easy. You know what you found, and you just have to put it down. The big choices are what to present and how to present it. Again, you can use yourself as a guide. What would you want to know if you were the reader? If this were a clinical study, you would want to know as much about the populations as possible. A table of their demographic characteristics would be in order. You surely want to know the results, so a table of means and variance (standard errors or standard deviations) or a figure of the raw data and means is necessary. You might want to know how variable 1 relates to variable 2, so provide either tables of correlation coefficients or scatter plots. And, you would like to know the results of statistical tests (p values, F, dF, etc.). Tables and figures should have legends with enough information so that they can be understood without reference to the text. The text merely says in words what is in the figures and tables. That part is easy.

4.2.4.4 *Discussion*

This is the most difficult section to write because it is somewhat unstructured and allows the author to put his findings in context. For the same reason, it is usually the most interesting, aside from the data themselves. In this section, you discuss the study and its implications. You should not simply restate the results. You should discuss any problems, limitations, or special features of the study. You should comment on the relationship between your findings and those of others and on any differences that exist. Identification of areas requiring further research or experimental implications of the findings should be discussed. Finally, some comment might be given regarding implications of the study that relate to broader issues in science or society. In short, the discussion section is the place for you to indicate what you think your study means.

4.2.4.5 *Afterwards*

Mailing the paper off gives you breathing time; however, you are not yet done. Editors and reviewers are now set to work. Generally, the editor-in-chief skims the paper and sends it off to the member of the editorial board most expert in the topic of the paper. That editor, in turn, either reads the paper in detail, requests reviews from two or more "experts" in the field, or does both. The "experts" can be people the editor knows and trusts, people prominent in the literature in the area of your paper, or people cited in your paper's bibliography. Some journals even request a list of possible reviewers from the author.

The journal usually sends the reviewer two forms. The first is for the editor's eyes alone. It requests specific recommendations, often in the form of checklists, for acceptance without revision, with minor revision, with major revision, or for rejection. The form provides for rating as good, fair, or poor the adequacy of the data, methods, discussion, presentation, and literature citation … in short, everything you wrote. Comments on appropriateness for the journal and on adherence to the format of the journal may also be requested, and space for special comments to the editor is also provided.

The second form, the one you see, is for comments for the authors. The format varies with the reviewer but most forms briefly summarize the major point of the paper, just so you and the editor know that the reviewer really read it, and then a tabulation of comments and criticisms. This requires that the reviewer carefully read and think about your paper, but reviewers are picked because they are productive and they are productive because they are busy working. While most do try to do reviews in a timely manner, your manuscript is generally not their top priority and the delay in getting to your paper accounts for a good deal of the delay in production. Almost all journals exhort their reviewers to return reviews within three weeks to a month and remind reviewers frequently thereafter and/or seek alternative reviewers. The quickest way to get your paper published is to write a perfect paper. Obviously, a paper that is so bad that it can be directly dismissed or so good that it requires no comment will be reviewed more quickly than one that requires more work because of marginal merit or poor language. The better the paper, the faster you get it back.

With all reviews in hand, the editor must make a decision. That decision is simple if all reviewers agree. The editor either returns the reviews with instructions, if the paper is accepted, or returns the reviews, a polite letter, and the manuscript, if it is not. When reviewers differ on whether a paper merits acceptance, editors may seek other opinions or make the choice themselves.

4.2.4.5.1 Acceptance.   Revision, or more work. Your joy at acceptance is diminished by the inane comments made by the reviewers about your magnificent manuscript and the letter directing you to revise your paper in accordance with those comments. Before you explode in rage or droop in despair, remember that the reviewer has volunteered precious time for the thankless task of detecting the weaknesses in your paper and suggesting improvements. The goal is to help you and to make for good science. The reviewer does not get a nickel for the task and has no motive to cause you sleepless nights. Give the comments careful consideration. You have been given free advice by experts, and it is only smart to heed what they say. If a reviewer misunderstood, it may be that your writing is misleading. Attend to it. If a reviewer disagrees with your interpretation, consider the arguments; however, consideration does not mean passive acceptance. Sometimes reviewers are simply wrong. You are entitled to say so in your return letter and to justify disregarding their advice or suggestions. In doing so, do not get cute and do not be sarcastic. Just present your arguments, remembering that they must be sufficiently compelling to convince the editor to overrule the reviewer.

The wheel turns. The revision starts the process anew. The editor again forwards it to the same reviewers, who return their reviews to the editor, who again writes to you, and around it goes until the work is sufficiently clean to merit publication. Usually, it takes a single turn.

4.2.4.5.2 Rejection.   The reviewers were not out to get you no matter what you believe, so do not be too discouraged. Journals reject many worthwhile articles that do not quite fit their orientation or standards. Look carefully at the reviews. Try to objectively reassess the adequacy of the data, the clarity of the writing, and the soundness of the conclusions. If you find them satisfactory, reformat the manuscript and send it off to another journal. If, on the other hand, you find the objections valid and new experiments are necessary, do them before submitting elsewhere. Besides building a bibliography, you are also building a reputation, and it is better to build one on good rather than mediocre work.

4.2.4.5.3 Caveat. All of the above discussion is directed toward today's printed journals. Increasingly, journals are going electronic. What this means for authors is still unclear. Certainly the lag between completing a study and distributing the results will be somewhat shortened. Many journals now accept papers in ASCII format on disk as well as on paper, but they still have to be written. Reviews return to editorial offices faster by FAX and e-mail than by regular mail, but they still must be reviewed by busy people. Electronic distribution may, however, significantly shorten the time between acceptance of a manuscript and its publication. Today that lag is about 6 months at best. Publication of a paper in a small journal with a set publication date may be quicker than in large journals limited by the number of articles that can be printed in an issue and the volume of acceptable papers. In principle, at least, electronic publication may make results available as quickly as papers are approved. While it may go faster, the approval process itself is likely to stay much the same.

The format requirements for most journals can be accessed on the Internet by using the name of the journal with almost any search engine. However, some journals, such as *Cell* and *Science*, have such general titles that unless you put quotes around the name, you will get lots of irrelevant material. Even with the quotes, you may get swamped and have to include "NOT" terms to exclude what you do not want. Links to the format requirements of some 3500 biomedical journals can be found on the web at:

http://www.mco.edu/lib/instr/libinsta.html

The International Committee of Medical Journal Editors (ICMJE) has been trying to establish uniform journal guidelines. In 1997, some 500 journals agreed to that format and the number has since grown. These uniform requirements can be accessed at:

http://www.cma.ca/mwc/uniform.htm

4.3 How to write a grant

4.3.1 Story

The results of the pilot study were terrific, and you were very excited. But your seed money will not last long and is certainly insufficient to carry out the main project. Also, you need additional supplies and personnel. But where to get the resources? Well, that was months ago, and, after failing to find any local source of money, you picked a funding agency out of a list gathered from the library and from that commercial firm. Finally, you got the courage to call the agency for a set of application forms and were lulled by the sultry-voiced assurances that your project was in the area of their interests and funding priorities. So you went to work. For two long months you wrote and rewrote and you gathered and filled out all the institutional approval forms for subjects and isotopes. Persuading your friends to read the grant and tear it apart was almost as difficult as writing it. Most of your friends skimmed the application, smiled, and told you how nice it was. That was fine for your ego but did not help. Only Abel and Cain took you at your word and tore it to pieces before gingerly handing it back to you. It was appalling how many inconsistencies they found and how many parts, so clear to you, left them confused. And so you smiled over clenched teeth and frantically spent another month rewriting the proposal. Finally, it made you physically ill just to look at it. Two days before the deadline you sighed "enough" and sent it off. Then the long wait began.

Now your grant, dog-eared and wrinkled, lies among others in a disheveled pile before your primary reviewer, Bob Brain. He is a big, broad man and an expert in the area of your grant, which is why he was selected to review it. But now he does not look like an expert. He looks like a tired, middle-aged man, which is what he is. His suit is wrinkled, his tie crooked, his face poorly shaved, and his little pig eyes are red-rimmed. He did not get much sleep on the airplane last night as it bounced through a storm, and he did not get to the hotel until nearly daylight. He had been too busy to come earlier. He did not get much sleep before that, either. The last two months were spent in writing his own grant application to cover the salary of the postdoc he invited to come from Tibet before realizing the money he set aside for that salary had somehow disappeared in the Administration's computer. Last week he was busy alternately reading grants, giving lectures, and trying to get a commitment from the administration to either find the money or cover the Tibetan's salary in case his grant is unfunded, preferably both.

The administrators, like most administrators, smiled but made no commitments.

No, he is not in a great mood. Bob is normally a nice fellow, even a jolly one given to folksy jokes, but today he is frustrated and tired. Around him the other members of the committee are slowly settling in. His friend Carl Corticoid, the group's expert in endocrinology, walks over and looks at him with a concerned expression on his long face.

"My God, Bob, you look awful. Just fly in?"

"Early this morning."

"You need some coffee, that's what you need. Hit your adenosine receptors, jack up your intracellular calcium, and inhibit your phosphodiesterase. That'll get you up. It's gonna be a long session. Shall I get you some?"

"No, thanks, I'll get it myself. It's a good idea. I need it."

Bob gets up and walks to the coffee urn, nodding and saying a few words to the other members of the committee. Only 10 of the 12 are there. The executive secretary is talking to the committee chairman, old Zachery Zingo, who at 64 is still producing more than 35-year-old Alex Abel, who is a department chairman and the youngest member of the committee. The committee members are a bright group of productive leaders in their fields. Bob respects them all, and a few are even friends. Perhaps Sam Shark is the most difficult to like. He has a smooth face, slick hair, a toothy smile, and a hard, slick mind. Maybe it is because he is still relatively young and unsure of his status that he is so aggressive and critical. He treats grant review like a game, with the prize going to the one who can find the most flaws. Whatever the reason, he is an unpleasant person. But he is smart, no question of that.

Bob sighs. He is first up, and your grant is the first to be reviewed. Bob wishes it were last. Everybody is fresh and eager for the first grant and does not yet feel the press of time. The first grant gets a thorough examination and lots of questions. By the time the last application comes up, it is late and everyone is so exhausted it gets a quick review. It would be easier to start with a poor application that everyone could chew up a bit before getting down to work. But yours is a good one. Bob had read it carefully three times during the past week, late at night and early in the morning, and could find only trivial problems, but it is always more difficult to defend than attack, and, of course, he could have missed some critical flaw that one of the others will pick up. Someone like Sammy Shark. Bob hopes not. He still has enough ego not to want to look like a fool. Yes, everyone is going to ask some questions, and Sammy Shark looks raring to go. Even those who only skimmed the grant will be trying to think up questions. From where he is standing, Bob can see three or four of them intently reading the abstract then skipping to the specific aims section. Well, the abstract of your grant summarizes the background for the proposal, the specific aims, the long-term goals, the general approach, and the significance of the research so concisely and neatly that even administrators can understand, appreciate, and use it when they set up the funding. And the specific aims section is well written, also; tight, clear "to…" statements. No rambling, no ambiguities, just statements such as "to determine…" and "to relate… ." The paper has a straight, clear listing of goals which are all consistent with the hypothesis, also specific and written to clearly indicate predicted directions of change.

The last two members hurry in, discussing problems about luggage on planes.

"Sorry we're late," said Roberta Receptor, the molecular biologist, "but our cab got stuck in traffic."

The chairman, Zachery Zingo, looks at his watch, which shows three minutes after the hour, nods, and says, "Okay, let's get started. We have a lot of work to do."

People move to the table, chairs scrape, coffee cups are set aside, papers shuffle, and the chairman picks up the schedule. He looks at Bob. "You're up," he says.

Bob picks up your grant and his yellow pad of notes. "This is a proposal to…," he begins, outlining the major goals of the project and then continuing through the experiments, one-by-one, showing how they are supposed to relate to the goals. Then comes the critique.

"This is a generally well-written proposal, and the studies outlined are likely to produce results commensurate with the goals. There are some ambiguities, however. The author does not make clear what he will do if experiment 3 does not come out as predicted. Presumably he will take it to mean… and will…, but this is not clearly spelled out." His voice drones on, making comments about other ambiguities, one in the demographics of subject selection, another in the selection of methods, and still another in assumptions about variance. At last, he concludes, "Despite these minor problems, this is a well-considered application in an area of some significance. It has a very good chance of filling an important gap in our knowledge, and I recommend it be approved with high priority."

"What about the budget?" asks Monty Money, the executive secretary. Monty taught psychology at a major university before he decided to go into grant administration.

"Well, it may be a little inflated but not much. The major piece of apparatus requested should not cost as much as the budget indicates unless prices have risen since last I looked. The technical help he is asking for seems reasonable. Subject costs seem high. It could probably be cut 5%."

There is a moment's pause, then Karen Klever says, "I'm second reviewer on this grant, and I really don't have much to add. I do agree it is well written and important and should be approved with high priority. I have some questions, however, one of which I'm really not competent to evaluate." She turns to Nathan Numbers, the statistician on the team. "Does the calculation for the number of subjects needed seem right to you? His estimate of variance for this kind of measure seems high, and I would think he could get away with fewer subjects."

Nathan Numbers looks at the section on data analysis for a moment and flips through the methods section until he finds the right place. His voice, as always, is so low everyone has to strain to hear. "Well, the estimate may be a bit high, but, in this case, it is certainly better to be high than to be low. It doesn't look as if he will have trouble getting enough subjects, and, if he has too few, the results may not reach statistical significance, and he will merely add another 'this-may-be-negative-but-I-don't-really-know' paper to the literature. I'm more bothered by the use of raw data for some of these calculations. Many biological variables do not have a normal distribution so that using standard statistical tests based on Gaussian distributions may produce misleading results. He probably should use log or square-root transformations of the raw data and test for normalcy before doing some of these calculations."

"But everyone uses this kind of raw data," objects Sam Shark, who always used the raw measures in his calculations.

Nathan looks at him without expression. "Then everyone may be wrong," he whispers and turns back to Karen. "It probably isn't critical in this case, because the measures are secondary to the major issue addressed, but you might include the suggestion in the 'pink sheet.'"

Bob and Karen nod, then Karen continues: "While he says he will randomize populations across treatments, he does not say who will do the randomizing. Presumably, it will be the assistant he is asking for and who is blind to all procedures. Finally, the intervals he is using to test interval reliability seem a bit long. Again, these are not critical to the study, and I concur in recommending approval."

Then the questions begin. Sam Shark leads the way: "The study depends on compliance. How is he going to assure that?"

Bob interrupts, "He can tell from the urinary measures."

Sam Shark frowns. "Well, maybe... ." He pauses. "But he doesn't say that in the grant."

Dean Doctor asks, "Does he say how any untoward effects will be handled?" Dean had only skimmed the grant, having enough trouble reading in detail the ones assigned to him.

"Yes, he outlines that on page 8."

Dean turns to page 8 and skims the section. He nods.

"The literature review is pretty skimpy," grunts Sam Shark.

"It seems pretty pointed and adequate to me," says Edward Eager. Edward had tangled with Sam before and there was little love lost between them. "Did he miss one of yours?"

Sam ignores him and continues, "The timetable seems overly optimistic."

"It probably is, but it seems to me that any timetable, especially in a fairly new area, is something of a fantasy, and if he misses a point, he is still likely to finish the study in the time requested."

Sam persists, "It seems to me that some of the methods are dated. There are more efficient ways to do some of these things now."

"You're right," Bob acknowledges, "but he has experience with those methods and they work in his hands. While we might suggest that he update some of them, the methods he lists will still get him where he wants to go."

And so it goes for another 15 minutes. But it becomes clear that those who have read your grant have no major questions, and those who have not have questions that are easily answered. Finally, there is a pause.

"No more questions?" asks Zack, looking around the table. No one says anything. "Okay, let's vote."

Each member picks up a small piece of paper, writes a number from 1 to 5 on it (with 1 being best), folds it, and drops it into a bowl. An assistant takes the bowl to Monty Money and together they add up the numbers while the study section continues. There are nine "1s" and three "2s" for a total of 15, or a mean score of 1.25. A good score, likely to get funded depending on the scores of the other grants and the total money assigned to the section.

Zack nods to Sam Shark, who is first reviewer on the next grant. Sam smiles.

"This is a grant by someone who does not know where he is going and cannot get there from here," he begins. "The specific aims are vague and poorly defined, the experiments are likely to give ambiguous results, and the results, even if they come out the way predicted, will not answer the question asked. It is a clinical study comparing patients with controls, but the control group selected is made up of hospital personnel who do not control for anything but age and sex. Any population differences found in the particular variables selected could as easily be due to differences in diet, drugs, activity levels, or sleep patterns. None of these possibilities is discussed.

"The background and significance section is wholly inadequate. It is not clear why the applicant wants to do this study, and his literature survey conveniently leaves out the literature that contradicts the findings he takes to support his hypothesis. Further, the aims stated here are not the same as those listed under the specific aims section, so it is not clear what his goals really are. The patient population he wishes to examine is fairly rare, and he provides no data on recruitment procedures or admission rates to indicate he will have enough patients to carry out the study if he gets the funds. Nor does he provide an estimate of the population size he needs to obtain statistical significance.

"Inclusion and exclusion criteria are inadequate. Part of this is a drug study, but he has not excluded subjects with liver or kidney disease. He does not consider possible untoward effects and does not state how they will be handled or who is responsible. The behavioral measures he proposes to use are his own and neither their validity nor reliability have been established. Nor is there anything in the grant suggesting they will attempt to establish either. Tissues will be assayed for several compounds but one of the procedures to be used lacks the specificity necessary in this case, and a second is too insensitive to pick up compounds at the level they exist in the tissues to be studied. The section on data analysis is ill considered. The author states he will do multiple T-tests but seems unaware that the number of variables to be compared by this procedure is so large he cannot rule out chance differences and false positives. Further, only some of the data are parametric, and he doesn't say how he will treat the rest.

"Finally, the budget. It is wholly inadequate. There is just no way to carry out this kind of study with this budget, unless he has some additional source of funds, which he does not identify. It is simply unrealistic. Indeed, if it were good enough to fund and we did fund it at this level, he would be unable to carry it out. In short, this is a poor grant, poorly written, badly conceived, and I move it be rejected."

"As secondary reviewer, even though the grant does have some merits, I tend to agree," says Paul Pleasant. Sam Shark snorts, but Paul continued. "It does address an important problem, although the approach is wholly inadequate. Rather than reject it outright, I would move for approval with very low priority and a very long pink sheet in the hope that it will stimulate the applicant to think a bit more critically and come back with a better proposal."

And the argument over the relative value of outright rejection vs. minimal approval goes on until a vote is taken (approval with a final priority score of 4.99) and the next review starts.

4.3.2 *Reality*

4.3.2.1 *Writing the grant*

This little fantasy about the workings of a study section is a parody of those used by the U.S. National Institutes of Health and exaggerates the review process. But, while different agencies use different numbers of reviewers in different combinations, the essential process is similar to that in the parody, and nearly all reviewers look for the same things. Almost all research applications require the same information, albeit in different forms, namely:

    I. Title
   II. Abstract (or summary)
  III. Specific aims (or hypotheses, objectives, or goals)
  IV. Background of the project and status of the field
   V. Significance of the project (sometimes combined with IV)
  VI. Research design and relationship of the studies to III
 VII. Methods (sometimes incorporated in VI)
VIII. Data analysis (sometimes incorporated in VI)
  IX. Budget and justification
   X. Such various administrative matters as a listing of personnel and their backgrounds, a timetable, and institutional approvals from human protection committees, animal protection committees, isotope committees, etc.

As indicated in our parody, your job is to clearly show the committee the importance of your project, the validity of your approach, and your competence to carry it out. The reviewer's job is to identify the proposal's strengths and weaknesses. The committee's job is to compare proposals.

Only a few suggestions can be made regarding how you might do your job. Most should be evident from the scenario above. To reiterate some of the most important "do's and don'ts," though:

1. *Do* aim for brevity, clarity, and specificity. Avoid redundancy. *Do not* use jargon, especially local jargon. Minimize the use of acronyms and, if you must use them, list them in an appendix.

2. *Do not* assume that the reviewers know the details of your field and procedures. They probably do, but detail them anyway.

3. *Do* give yourself a reasonable time to prepare the grant application. Solicit critical reviews by others and incorporate relevant comments into the grant before it is sent out. If the whole application is to be written fresh and you cannot lift sections from previous applications, give yourself at least 2 to 3 months.

4. *Do* give thought to the title and abstract. They are the only items you can be sure will be read by all reviewers and grant administrators. Some large agencies also use them to select the experts who will review the application. The title should be complete. The abstract should state the general problem, as well as its social, medical, or scientific significance, your approach, and the significance of the expected results.

5. *Do* make specific aims (hypotheses, objectives, goals) specific. When possible, number them, and phrase them as "to..." statements, such as "to determine if fluctuations in blood serotonin predict suicidal attempts" or "to compare the effects of psychotherapy and fluoxetine on suicidal ideation." If hypotheses are requested, make them specific and identify the direction of any changes or differences you hypothesize (e.g., 1. Increased fluctuations in blood serotonin predict suicidal attempts; 2. Psychotherapy will be more effective than fluoxetine in preventing suicidal ideation). Maintain consistency in aims throughout the application. Reviewers become unhappy if the implied or stated goals in the specific aims section differ from those in another section.

6. *Do* cite your own preliminary studies, if you have them, as well as the basis for your interest in the problem, in the background section. *Do* cite all sides of the relevant literature specifically related to your proposal and try to reconcile any conflicts bearing on your study or explain how they will not affect it. *Do* keep it brief (two to three pages).

7. *Do* be brief but make the strongest case you can for the economic, social, health, or scientific importance of the proposal if there is a significance section. Data supporting such arguments can often be obtained from governmental agencies and from yearly almanacs of data. This section is increasingly important as funding declines.

8. *Do* make sure the experiments are commensurate with the goals in the research design section. *Do* mention and briefly discuss alternative outcomes. *Do* detail the sequence of procedures. This is especially important in clinical studies where you should define who will do what when. An outline of procedures or experiments is often helpful.

9. *Do* make sure that the methods listed in the methods section work and are of sufficient sensitivity and specificity to meet your needs.

10. *Do* consult a statistician on both research design and data analysis if you are using a complex design with parametric and nonparametric data. If not, *do* state how you calculated the number of subjects you need and how the data will be treated.

11. *Do* be realistic when writing the budget and justification. Some inflation to cover real costs you did not consider is expected. Grants are seldom rejected because of a modestly inflated budget, although the excess might be cut. *Do not* ask for less than you need. First, doing so reflects on your judgment. Second, if you get the grant, you may be unable to carry it out. Just as grants are not rejected because of slightly inflated budgets, they may not be accepted because of a deflated one.

E.R. Oetting listed ten fatal mistakes in writing a grant:

1. Writing a grant to get support for a treatment program
2. Proposing work outside your area of competence
3. Providing insufficient detail
4. Ignoring previous recommendations in reviews
5. Proposing to develop a scale without adequately defining the scale, the need, or the methods

6. Simply tacking onto the disease-of-the-week
7. The no-problem problem
8. Explaining why a critical part of the study cannot be done
9. Using inappropriate tests or measures
10. Not applying

Avoid them.

4.3.2.2 *Afterwards*

The grant has been reviewed and the committee has made its decisions. Now what? The hidden process cranks on. Review committees are usually advisory to funding committees, which have the job of matching scientific excellence with agency goals and available funding. Sometimes they also adjudicate between the recommendations of several review panels, political directives, and social forces.

While funding committees usually follow the recommendations of their review panels, applications of lesser scientific value may be funded out of order because of special relevance to agency goals. For example, agencies devoted to the conquest of a specific disease might fund a less rigorous clinical study offering the possibility of immediate application over a scientifically better preclinical one of more uncertain relevance. Special political or social factors may also color funding, especially for agencies subject to political overview. At times, agencies or governments may solicit grants directed to particular social or political problems which may be separately or preferentially funded over scientifically better ones in other areas. Unfortunately, political or social considerations may also, on rare occasions, prevent government or agency funding of some lines of investigation regardless of their scientific merit or importance.

Whether the grant is funded or not, you will eventually receive a letter and a critique that will set you back to work. Typically, the substantive part of the critique is written by its primary reviewer with input from the committee secretary and the committee chairman. How you read it depends somewhat on whether the grant is approved and funded, approved but not funded, or not approved.

The critique of an approved and funded grant should be taken as free expert opinion and advice. Focus particularly on discussions of the strengths of the grant with secondary attention to the most important problems. For three reasons it is generally more efficient to attend to and productively exploit the strengths of the proposal than to spend significant time or resources redressing more minor weaknesses. First, the strengths of the proposal impressed the committee more than its defects; otherwise, it would not have been funded. Second, the composition of the review panel will likely change by the time of renewal and a second committee may not concentrate on the same defects as the first. Third, changes in the field may make old defects moot.

If the grant is approved but not funded, the reading may be more difficult. Ideally, critiques should explicitly identify weaknesses and should provide real reasons justifying the priority score. Sometimes, however, they provide weak good reasons for real reasons and it is important that you distinguish between them. Increasingly, very good applications are not funded because of insufficient money. While authors want to regard all critiques as unreasonable or trivial, if critiques are clear, directed at specific and relevant issues, and even seem justified, rejoice at good news hidden in the bad news. The application might receive funding if the defects can be corrected. Your task is to correct them. That might be very difficult but at least the goal is clear. During the process, all issues raised in the critique must be addressed. The resubmitted application will very likely go to the same review panel and the same primary reviewer. Even if it is sent to another review panel, the critique will follow and answers will be sought.

On the other hand, if the comments really do seem to be trivial, irrelevant, and vague, watch out. The message may not be in the words themselves. Vagueness may be due to literary weakness but generally is not. Most often the real reasons cannot be easily explicated and good reasons are substituted instead. This most commonly occurs with "so what" applications in which a proposed work may be methodologically sound but, in the committee's view, is conceptually dull, scientifically unimportant, or irrelevant to the pressing issues of the day as compared to other applications. Because it is difficult to justify a critique which simply says "who cares," the review instead is comprised of carping comments about minor details, irrelevancies, and general statements. In such a case, simply revising the grant to address these minor details will do no good. It simply wastes time. At the least, any revision should contain a stronger justification and presentation of the potential significance of the results as well as answering all the comments one can. Sometimes nothing will help. A call and frank questions to the secretary of the review section may often confirm a suspicion and save the work of a revision. A more expensive indicator of the substitution of good reasons for real reasons is the return of a revised application with an entirely different set of criticisms and a still lower priority score.

Other classes of grants that may elicit ambiguous critiques are the "me, too" variety, conceptually indistinguishable replicas of each other; "wheel" grants seemingly aimed at rediscovering what is already well established; and "dust bowl" grants, which continue to plow thoroughly gleaned fields. If you suspect your grant might have been mistaken for one of these, rewrite it to emphasize its unique, new, and imaginative features.

Grants are reviewed by humans, thus the process suffers from human frailties ranging from unconscious jealousy through unconscious plagiarism to failures of intelligence and imagination. As an applicant, you can do little about these except to write as clearly as possible and present supporting data for your approach. This is particularly true if the material is truly innovative, for the review process is generally better at assessing competence than genius, as witnessed by the many Nobelists whose innovations were at first rejected by their peers. The clearer the concepts, the sharper the writing, the better your data, and the more important the problem and its implications, the better you will fare.

Good luck!

4.4 Web sites

The increase in grant funding has resulted in the growth of commercial sites offering grant information. These are not listed because their life span in uncertain. Some universities also offer information on granting services; some charge a fee. Most can be accessed from search engines using the terms "research grants," "biomedical research grants," or "biomedical research granting agencies." The search is sometimes improved on in some search engines by inserting "+" or "and" between words. Naming the agency or charity in most search engine windows will produce its home page. Many will download their grant application forms. One general address permitting direct contact with some private granting agencies is

http://www.socialpsychology.org/grants.htm.

Almost every government lists grants. Below are listed a few from the U.S.; others can be obtained by searching under the name of the institute.

U.S. National Institutes of Health (NIH):

http://grants.nih.gov/grants/
http://grants.nih.gov/grants/policy/policy.htm
http://grants.nih.gov/grants/forms.htm

U.S. National Institute of Mental Health (NIHM):

http://www.nimh.nih.gov/grants/nihgrants.cfn

U.S. National Science Foundation (NSF):

http://www.nsf.gov/home/grants.htm

Bibliography

Dennis, M., Ferguson, B., and Tyrer, P., Rating instruments in research methods, in *Psychiatry: A Beginner's Guide*, Freeman C. and Tyrer, P., Eds., Gaskell Press, 1995, p. 83.

Department of Clinical Epidemiology and Biostatistics, McMaster University Health Science Center, Clinical epidemiology rounds: how to read clinical journals. 1. Why to read them and how to start reading them critically, *Canad. J. Med.*, 124, 555, 1981.

Department of Clinical Epidemiology and Biostatistics, McMaster University Health Science Center, Clinical epidemiology rounds: how to read clinical journals. 2. To learn about a diagnostic test, *Canad. J. Med.*, 124, 703, 1981.

Department of Clinical Epidemiology and Biostatistics, McMaster University Health Science Center, Clinical epidemiology rounds: how to read clinical journals. 3. To learn the clinical course and prognosis of disease, *Canad. J. Med.*, 124, 869 1981.

Department of Clinical Epidemiology and Biostatistics, McMaster University Health Science Center, Clinical epidemiology rounds: how to read clinical journals. 4. To determine etiology or causation, *Canad. J. Med.*, 124, 985, 1981.

Department of Clinical Epidemiology and Biostatistics, McMaster University Health Science Center, Clinical epidemiology rounds: how to read clinical journals. 5. To distinguish useful from useless or even harmful therapy, *Canad. J. Med.*, 124, 1156, 1981.

Fava, A. and Rosenbaum J.F., Research designs and methods in psychiatry, in *Techniques in the Behavioral and Neural Sciences*, Vol. 9, Houston, J.P., Ed., New York, Elsivier, 1992.

Hamilton, M., A rating scale for depression, *J. Neurol. Neurosurg. Psychiat.*, 23, 56, 1960.

Hopkins, C.G. and Cole, S.W., A contribution to the chemistry of proteides. Part I. A preliminary study of a hitherto undescribed product of tryptic digestion, *J. Physiol.*, 27, 418, 1901–1902.

Kramer, M., A discussion of the concepts of incidence and prevalence as related to epidemiological studies of mental disorders, *Amer. J. Public Health*, 47, 826, 1957.

Murphy, S. and Tyrer, P., Rating scales for special purposes. I. Psychotherapy, in *Research Methods in Psychiatry: A Beginner's Guide*, Freeman, C. and Tyrer, P., Eds., Gaskell Press, 1995, p. 83.

Oetting, E.R., Ten fatal mistakes in grant writing, *Professional Psychology: Research and Practice*, 17, 570, 1986.

Overall, J.E. and Gorham, D.R., The brief psychiatric rating scale, *Psychol. Reports*, 10, 799, 1962.

Reigelhaupt, L.M., Investigation of urinary excretion patterns in psychotic subjects, *J. Nerv. Ment. Dis.*, 127, 22, 1958.

Spitzer, R.L., Williams, J.B.W., Gibbon, M., and First, M.B., *Structured Clinical Interview for DSM-III* (including User's Guide), American Psychiatric Press, Washington, D.C., 1990.

Tsuang M.T. and Winokur, G., The Iowa 500: field work in a 35-year follow-up of depression, mania, and schizophrenia, *Canad. Psychiat. Assoc. J.*, 20, 359, 1975.

Tyrer, P. and Murphy, S., Rating scales for special purposes. II. Complex subjects, in *Research Methods in Psychiatry: A Beginner's Guide*, Freeman, C. and Tyrer, P., Eds., Gaskell Press, 1995, pp. 273–295.

Index